Mometrix

TEST PREPARATION

CCCN®

Exam Secrets Study Guide

Dear Future Exam Success Story

First of all, **THANK YOU** for purchasing Mometrix study materials!

Second, congratulations! You are one of the few determined test-takers who are committed to doing whatever it takes to excel on your exam. **You have come to the right place.** We developed these study materials with one goal in mind: to deliver you the information you need in a format that's concise and easy to use.

In addition to optimizing your guide for the content of the test, we've outlined our recommended steps for breaking down the preparation process into small, attainable goals so you can make sure you stay on track.

We've also analyzed the entire test-taking process, identifying the most common pitfalls and showing how you can overcome them and be ready for any curveball the test throws you.

Standardized testing is one of the biggest obstacles on your road to success, which only increases the importance of doing well in the high-pressure, high-stakes environment of test day. Your results on this test could have a significant impact on your future, and this guide provides the information and practical advice to help you achieve your full potential on test day.

Your success is our success

We would love to hear from you! If you would like to share the story of your exam success or if you have any questions or comments in regard to our products, please contact us at **800-673-8175** or **support@mometrix.com**.

Thanks again for your business and we wish you continued success!

Sincerely,
The Mometrix Test Preparation Team

TABLE OF CONTENTS

Introduction

Thank you for purchasing this resource! You have made the choice to prepare yourself for a test that could have a huge impact on your future, and this guide is designed to help you be fully ready for test day. Obviously, it's important to have a solid understanding of the test material, but you also need to be prepared for the unique environment and stressors of the test, so that you can perform to the best of your abilities.

For this purpose, the first section that appears in this guide is the **Secret Keys**. We've devoted countless hours to meticulously researching what works and what doesn't, and we've boiled down our findings to the five most impactful steps you can take to improve your performance on the test. We start at the beginning with study planning and move through the preparation process, all the way to the testing strategies that will help you get the most out of what you know when you're finally sitting in front of the test.

We recommend that you start preparing for your test as far in advance as possible. However, if you've bought this guide as a last-minute study resource and only have a few days before your test, we recommend that you skip over the first two Secret Keys since they address a long-term study plan.

If you struggle with **test anxiety**, we strongly encourage you to check out our recommendations for how you can overcome it. Test anxiety is a formidable foe, but it can be beaten, and we want to make sure you have the tools you need to defeat it.

Secret Key #1 – Plan Big, Study Small

There's a lot riding on your performance. If you want to ace this test, you're going to need to keep your skills sharp and the material fresh in your mind. You need a plan that lets you review everything you need to know while still fitting in your schedule. We'll break this strategy down into three categories.

Information Organization

Start with the information you already have: the official test outline. From this, you can make a complete list of all the concepts you need to cover before the test. Organize these concepts into groups that can be studied together, and create a list of any related vocabulary you need to learn so you can brush up on any difficult terms. You'll want to keep this vocabulary list handy once you actually start studying since you may need to add to it along the way.

Time Management

Once you have your set of study concepts, decide how to spread them out over the time you have left before the test. Break your study plan into small, clear goals so you have a manageable task for each day and know exactly what you're doing. Then just focus on one small step at a time. When you manage your time this way, you don't need to spend hours at a time studying. Studying a small block of content for a short period each day helps you retain information better and avoid stressing over how much you have left to do. You can relax knowing that you have a plan to cover everything in time. In order for this strategy to be effective though, you have to start studying early and stick to your schedule. Avoid the exhaustion and futility that comes from last-minute cramming!

Study Environment

The environment you study in has a big impact on your learning. Studying in a coffee shop, while probably more enjoyable, is not likely to be as fruitful as studying in a quiet room. It's important to keep distractions to a minimum. You're only planning to study for a short block of time, so make the most of it. Don't pause to check your phone or get up to find a snack. It's also important to **avoid multitasking**. Research has consistently shown that multitasking will make your studying dramatically less effective. Your study area should also be comfortable and well-lit so you don't have the distraction of straining your eyes or sitting on an uncomfortable chair.

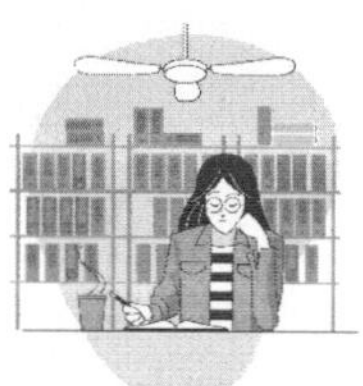

The time of day you study is also important. You want to be rested and alert. Don't wait until just before bedtime. Study when you'll be most likely to comprehend and remember. Even better, if you know what time of day your test will be, set that time aside for study. That way your brain will be used to working on that subject at that specific time and you'll have a better chance of recalling information.

Finally, it can be helpful to team up with others who are studying for the same test. Your actual studying should be done in as isolated an environment as possible, but the work of organizing the information and setting up the study plan can be divided up. In between study sessions, you can discuss with your teammates the concepts that you're all studying and quiz each other on the details. Just be sure that your teammates are as serious about the test as you are. If you find that your study time is being replaced with social time, you might need to find a new team.

Secret Key #2 – Make Your Studying Count

You're devoting a lot of time and effort to preparing for this test, so you want to be absolutely certain it will pay off. This means doing more than just reading the content and hoping you can remember it on test day. It's important to make every minute of study count. There are two main areas you can focus on to make your studying count.

Retention

It doesn't matter how much time you study if you can't remember the material. You need to make sure you are retaining the concepts. To check your retention of the information you're learning, try recalling it at later times with minimal prompting. Try carrying around flashcards and glance at one or two from time to time or ask a friend who's also studying for the test to quiz you.

To enhance your retention, look for ways to put the information into practice so that you can apply it rather than simply recalling it. If you're using the information in practical ways, it will be much easier to remember. Similarly, it helps to solidify a concept in your mind if you're not only reading it to yourself but also explaining it to someone else. Ask a friend to let you teach them about a concept you're a little shaky on (or speak aloud to an imaginary audience if necessary). As you try to summarize, define, give examples, and answer your friend's questions, you'll understand the concepts better and they will stay with you longer. Finally, step back for a big picture view and ask yourself how each piece of information fits with the whole subject. When you link the different concepts together and see them working together as a whole, it's easier to remember the individual components.

Finally, practice showing your work on any multi-step problems, even if you're just studying. Writing out each step you take to solve a problem will help solidify the process in your mind, and you'll be more likely to remember it during the test.

Modality

Modality simply refers to the means or method by which you study. Choosing a study modality that fits your own individual learning style is crucial. No two people learn best in exactly the same way, so it's important to know your strengths and use them to your advantage.

For example, if you learn best by visualization, focus on visualizing a concept in your mind and draw an image or a diagram. Try color-coding your notes, illustrating them, or creating symbols that will trigger your mind to recall a learned concept. If you learn best by hearing or discussing information, find a study partner who learns the same way or read aloud to yourself. Think about how to put the information in your own words. Imagine that you are giving a lecture on the topic and record yourself so you can listen to it later.

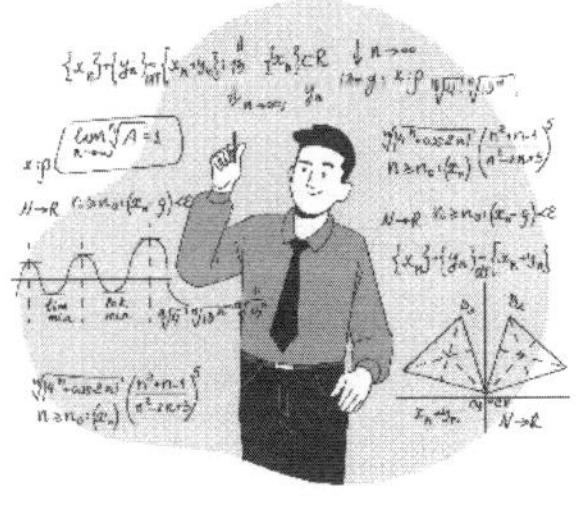

For any learning style, flashcards can be helpful. Organize the information so you can take advantage of spare moments to review. Underline key words or phrases. Use different colors for different categories. Mnemonic devices (such as creating a short list in which every item starts with the same letter) can also help with retention. Find what works best for you and use it to store the information in your mind most effectively and easily.

Secret Key #3 – Practice the Right Way

Your success on test day depends not only on how many hours you put into preparing, but also on whether you prepared the right way. It's good to check along the way to see if your studying is paying off. One of the most effective ways to do this is by taking practice tests to evaluate your progress. Practice tests are useful because they show exactly where you need to improve. Every time you take a practice test, pay special attention to these three groups of questions:

- The questions you got wrong
- The questions you had to guess on, even if you guessed right
- The questions you found difficult or slow to work through

This will show you exactly what your weak areas are, and where you need to devote more study time. Ask yourself why each of these questions gave you trouble. Was it because you didn't understand the material? Was it because you didn't remember the vocabulary? Do you need more repetitions on this type of question to build speed and confidence? Dig into those questions and figure out how you can strengthen your weak areas as you go back to review the material.

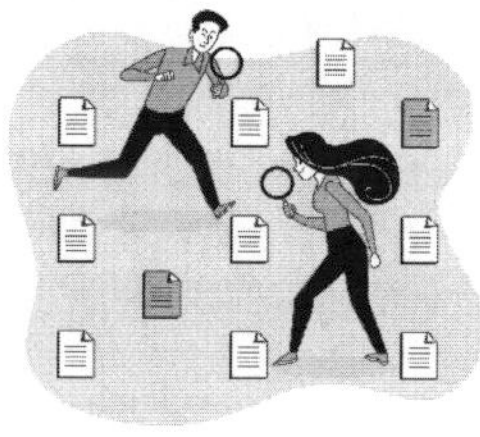

Additionally, many practice tests have a section explaining the answer choices. It can be tempting to read the explanation and think that you now have a good understanding of the concept. However, an explanation likely only covers part of the question's broader context. Even if the explanation makes perfect sense, **go back and investigate** every concept related to the question until you're positive you have a thorough understanding.

As you go along, keep in mind that the practice test is just that: practice. Memorizing these questions and answers will not be very helpful on the actual test because it is unlikely to have any of the same exact questions. If you only know the right answers to the sample questions, you won't be prepared for the real thing. **Study the concepts** until you understand them fully, and then you'll be able to answer any question that shows up on the test.

It's important to wait on the practice tests until you're ready. If you take a test on your first day of study, you may be overwhelmed by the amount of material covered and how much you need to learn. Work up to it gradually.

On test day, you'll need to be prepared for answering questions, managing your time, and using the test-taking strategies you've learned. It's a lot to balance, like a mental marathon that will have a big impact on your future. Like training for a marathon, you'll need to start slowly and work your way up. When test day arrives, you'll be ready.

Start with the strategies you've read in the first two Secret Keys—plan your course and study in the way that works best for you. If you have time, consider using multiple study resources to get different approaches to the same concepts. It can be helpful to see difficult concepts from more than one angle. Then find a good source for practice tests. Many times, the test website will suggest potential study resources or provide sample tests.

Practice Test Strategy

If you're able to find at least three practice tests, we recommend this strategy:

Untimed and Open-Book Practice

Take the first test with no time constraints and with your notes and study guide handy. Take your time and focus on applying the strategies you've learned.

Timed and Open-Book Practice

Take the second practice test open-book as well, but set a timer and practice pacing yourself to finish in time.

Timed and Closed-Book Practice

Take any other practice tests as if it were test day. Set a timer and put away your study materials. Sit at a table or desk in a quiet room, imagine yourself at the testing center, and answer questions as quickly and accurately as possible.

Keep repeating timed and closed-book tests on a regular basis until you run out of practice tests or it's time for the actual test. Your mind will be ready for the schedule and stress of test day, and you'll be able to focus on recalling the material you've learned.

Secret Key #4 – Pace Yourself

Once you're fully prepared for the material on the test, your biggest challenge on test day will be managing your time. Just knowing that the clock is ticking can make you panic even if you have plenty of time left. Work on pacing yourself so you can build confidence against the time constraints of the exam. Pacing is a difficult skill to master, especially in a high-pressure environment, so **practice is vital**.

Set time expectations for your pace based on how much time is available. For example, if a section has 60 questions and the time limit is 30 minutes, you know you have to average 30 seconds or less per question in order to answer them all. Although 30 seconds is the hard limit, set 25 seconds per question as your goal, so you reserve extra time to spend on harder questions. When you budget extra time for the harder questions, you no longer have any reason to stress when those questions take longer to answer.

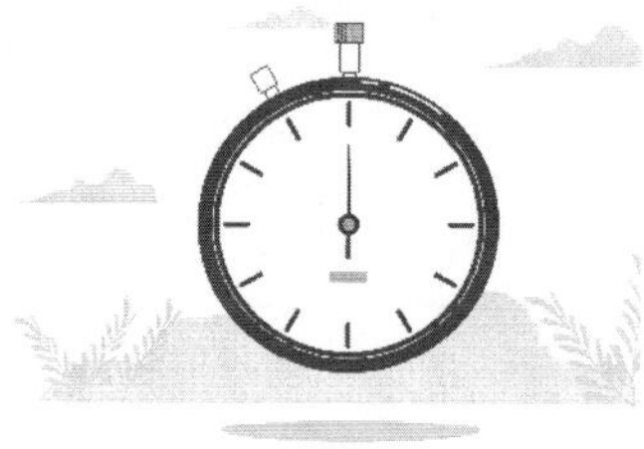

Don't let this time expectation distract you from working through the test at a calm, steady pace, but keep it in mind so you don't spend too much time on any one question. Recognize that taking extra time on one question you don't understand may keep you from answering two that you do understand later in the test. If your time limit for a question is up and you're still not sure of the answer, mark it and move on, and come back to it later if the time and the test format allow. If the testing format doesn't allow you to return to earlier questions, just make an educated guess; then put it out of your mind and move on.

On the easier questions, be careful not to rush. It may seem wise to hurry through them so you have more time for the challenging ones, but it's not worth missing one if you know the concept and just didn't take the time to read the question fully. Work efficiently but make sure you understand the question and have looked at all of the answer choices, since more than one may seem right at first.

Even if you're paying attention to the time, you may find yourself a little behind at some point. You should speed up to get back on track, but do so wisely. Don't panic; just take a few seconds less on each question until you're caught up. Don't guess without thinking, but do look through the answer choices and eliminate any you know are wrong. If you can get down to two choices, it is often worthwhile to guess from those. Once you've chosen an answer, move on and don't dwell on any that you skipped or had to hurry through. If a question was taking too long, chances are it was one of the harder ones, so you weren't as likely to get it right anyway.

On the other hand, if you find yourself getting ahead of schedule, it may be beneficial to slow down a little. The more quickly you work, the more likely you are to make a careless mistake that will affect your score. You've budgeted time for each question, so don't be afraid to spend that time. Practice an efficient but careful pace to get the most out of the time you have.

Secret Key #5 – Have a Plan for Guessing

When you're taking the test, you may find yourself stuck on a question. Some of the answer choices seem better than others, but you don't see the one answer choice that is obviously correct. What do you do?

The scenario described above is very common, yet most test takers have not effectively prepared for it. Developing and practicing a plan for guessing may be one of the single most effective uses of your time as you get ready for the exam.

In developing your plan for guessing, there are three questions to address:

- When should you start the guessing process?
- How should you narrow down the choices?
- Which answer should you choose?

When to Start the Guessing Process

Unless your plan for guessing is to select C every time (which, despite its merits, is not what we recommend), you need to leave yourself enough time to apply your answer elimination strategies. Since you have a limited amount of time for each question, that means that if you're going to give yourself the best shot at guessing correctly, you have to decide quickly whether or not you will guess.

Of course, the best-case scenario is that you don't have to guess at all, so first, see if you can answer the question based on your knowledge of the subject and basic reasoning skills. Focus on the key words in the question and try to jog your memory of related topics. Give yourself a chance to bring the knowledge to mind, but once you realize that you don't have (or you can't access) the knowledge you need to answer the question, it's time to start the guessing process.

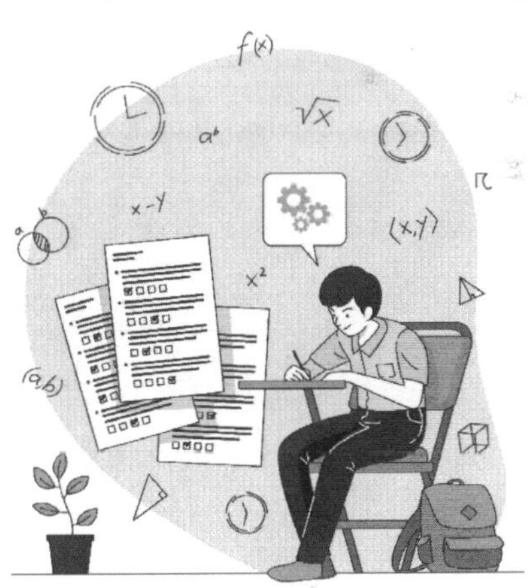

It's almost always better to start the guessing process too early than too late. It only takes a few seconds to remember something and answer the question from knowledge. Carefully eliminating wrong answer choices takes longer. Plus, going through the process of eliminating answer choices can actually help jog your memory.

Summary: Start the guessing process as soon as you decide that you can't answer the question based on your knowledge.

How to Narrow Down the Choices

The next chapter in this book (**Test-Taking Strategies**) includes a wide range of strategies for how to approach questions and how to look for answer choices to eliminate. You will definitely want to read those carefully, practice them, and figure out which ones work best for you. Here though, we're going to address a mindset rather than a particular strategy.

Your odds of guessing an answer correctly depend on how many options you are choosing from.

Number of options left	5	4	3	2	1
Odds of guessing correctly	20%	25%	33%	50%	100%

You can see from this chart just how valuable it is to be able to eliminate incorrect answers and make an educated guess, but there are two things that many test takers do that cause them to miss out on the benefits of guessing:

- Accidentally eliminating the correct answer
- Selecting an answer based on an impression

We'll look at the first one here, and the second one in the next section.

To avoid accidentally eliminating the correct answer, we recommend a thought exercise called **the $5 challenge**. In this challenge, you only eliminate an answer choice from contention if you are willing to bet $5 on it being wrong. Why $5? Five dollars is a small but not insignificant amount of money. It's an amount you could afford to lose but wouldn't want to throw away. And while losing $5 once might not hurt too much, doing it twenty times will set you back $100. In the same way, each small decision you make—eliminating a choice here, guessing on a question there—won't by itself impact your score very much, but when you put them all together, they can make a big difference. By holding each answer choice elimination decision to a higher standard, you can reduce the risk of accidentally eliminating the correct answer.

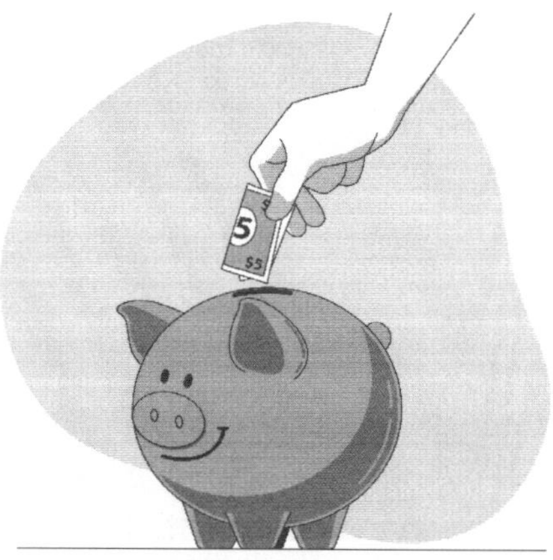

The $5 challenge can also be applied in a positive sense: If you are willing to bet $5 that an answer choice *is* correct, go ahead and mark it as correct.

Summary: Only eliminate an answer choice if you are willing to bet $5 that it is wrong.

Which Answer to Choose

You're taking the test. You've run into a hard question and decided you'll have to guess. You've eliminated all the answer choices you're willing to bet $5 on. Now you have to pick an answer. Why do we even need to talk about this? Why can't you just pick whichever one you feel like when the time comes?

The answer to these questions is that if you don't come into the test with a plan, you'll rely on your impression to select an answer choice, and if you do that, you risk falling into a trap. The test writers know that everyone who takes their test will be guessing on some of the questions, so they intentionally write wrong answer choices to seem plausible. You still have to pick an answer though, and if the wrong answer choices are designed to look right, how can you ever be sure that you're not falling for their trap? The best solution we've found to this dilemma is to take the decision out of your hands entirely. Here is the process we recommend:

Once you've eliminated any choices that you are confident (willing to bet $5) are wrong, select the first remaining choice as your answer.

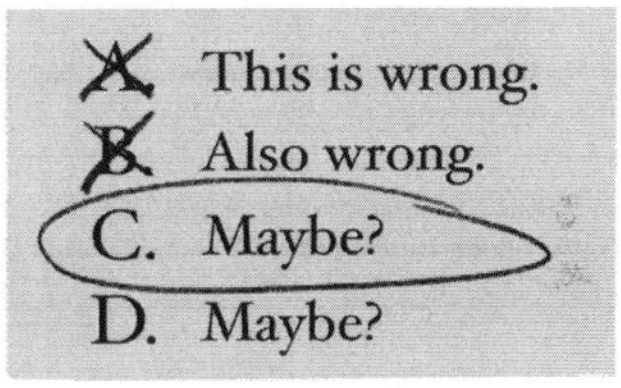

Whether you choose to select the first remaining choice, the second, or the last, the important thing is that you use some preselected standard. Using this approach guarantees that you will not be enticed into selecting an answer choice that looks right, because you are not basing your decision on how the answer choices look.

This is not meant to make you question your knowledge. Instead, it is to help you recognize the difference between your knowledge and your impressions. There's a huge difference between thinking an answer is right because of what you know, and thinking an answer is right because it looks or sounds like it should be right.

Summary: To ensure that your selection is appropriately random, make a predetermined selection from among all answer choices you have not eliminated.

Test-Taking Strategies

This section contains a list of test-taking strategies that you may find helpful as you work through the test. By taking what you know and applying logical thought, you can maximize your chances of answering any question correctly!

It is very important to realize that every question is different and every person is different: no single strategy will work on every question, and no single strategy will work for every person. That's why we've included all of them here, so you can try them out and determine which ones work best for different types of questions and which ones work best for you.

Question Strategies

✓ Read Carefully

Read the question and the answer choices carefully. Don't miss the question because you misread the terms. You have plenty of time to read each question thoroughly and make sure you understand what is being asked. Yet a happy medium must be attained, so don't waste too much time. You must read carefully and efficiently.

✓ Contextual Clues

Look for contextual clues. If the question includes a word you are not familiar with, look at the immediate context for some indication of what the word might mean. Contextual clues can often give you all the information you need to decipher the meaning of an unfamiliar word. Even if you can't determine the meaning, you may be able to narrow down the possibilities enough to make a solid guess at the answer to the question.

✓ Prefixes

If you're having trouble with a word in the question or answer choices, try dissecting it. Take advantage of every clue that the word might include. Prefixes can be a huge help. Usually, they allow you to determine a basic meaning. *Pre-* means before, *post-* means after, *pro-* is positive, *de-* is negative. From prefixes, you can get an idea of the general meaning of the word and try to put it into context.

✓ Hedge Words

Watch out for critical hedge words, such as *likely, may, can, often, almost, mostly, usually, generally, rarely*, and *sometimes*. Question writers insert these hedge phrases to cover every possibility. Often an answer choice will be wrong simply because it leaves no room for exception. Be on guard for answer choices that have definitive words such as *exactly* and *always*.

✓ Switchback Words

Stay alert for *switchbacks*. These are the words and phrases frequently used to alert you to shifts in thought. The most common switchback words are *but, although*, and *however*. Others include *nevertheless, on the other hand, even though, while, in spite of, despite*, and *regardless of*. Switchback words are important to catch because they can change the direction of the question or an answer choice.

⊘ FACE VALUE

When in doubt, use common sense. Accept the situation in the problem at face value. Don't read too much into it. These problems will not require you to make wild assumptions. If you have to go beyond creativity and warp time or space in order to have an answer choice fit the question, then you should move on and consider the other answer choices. These are normal problems rooted in reality. The applicable relationship or explanation may not be readily apparent, but it is there for you to figure out. Use your common sense to interpret anything that isn't clear.

Answer Choice Strategies

⊘ ANSWER SELECTION

The most thorough way to pick an answer choice is to identify and eliminate wrong answers until only one is left, then confirm it is the correct answer. Sometimes an answer choice may immediately seem right, but be careful. The test writers will usually put more than one reasonable answer choice on each question, so take a second to read all of them and make sure that the other choices are not equally obvious. As long as you have time left, it is better to read every answer choice than to pick the first one that looks right without checking the others.

⊘ ANSWER CHOICE FAMILIES

An answer choice family consists of two (in rare cases, three) answer choices that are very similar in construction and cannot all be true at the same time. If you see two answer choices that are direct opposites or parallels, one of them is usually the correct answer. For instance, if one answer choice says that quantity *x* increases and another either says that quantity *x* decreases (opposite) or says that quantity *y* increases (parallel), then those answer choices would fall into the same family. An answer choice that doesn't match the construction of the answer choice family is more likely to be incorrect. Most questions will not have answer choice families, but when they do appear, you should be prepared to recognize them.

⊘ ELIMINATE ANSWERS

Eliminate answer choices as soon as you realize they are wrong, but make sure you consider all possibilities. If you are eliminating answer choices and realize that the last one you are left with is also wrong, don't panic. Start over and consider each choice again. There may be something you missed the first time that you will realize on the second pass.

⊘ AVOID FACT TRAPS

Don't be distracted by an answer choice that is factually true but doesn't answer the question. You are looking for the choice that answers the question. Stay focused on what the question is asking for so you don't accidentally pick an answer that is true but incorrect. Always go back to the question and make sure the answer choice you've selected actually answers the question and is not merely a true statement.

⊘ EXTREME STATEMENTS

In general, you should avoid answers that put forth extreme actions as standard practice or proclaim controversial ideas as established fact. An answer choice that states the "process should be used in certain situations, if..." is much more likely to be correct than one that states the "process should be discontinued completely." The first is a calm rational statement and doesn't even make a definitive, uncompromising stance, using a hedge word *if* to provide wiggle room, whereas the second choice is far more extreme.

☑ Benchmark

As you read through the answer choices and you come across one that seems to answer the question well, mentally select that answer choice. This is not your final answer, but it's the one that will help you evaluate the other answer choices. The one that you selected is your benchmark or standard for judging each of the other answer choices. Every other answer choice must be compared to your benchmark. That choice is correct until proven otherwise by another answer choice beating it. If you find a better answer, then that one becomes your new benchmark. Once you've decided that no other choice answers the question as well as your benchmark, you have your final answer.

☑ Predict the Answer

Before you even start looking at the answer choices, it is often best to try to predict the answer. When you come up with the answer on your own, it is easier to avoid distractions and traps because you will know exactly what to look for. The right answer choice is unlikely to be word-for-word what you came up with, but it should be a close match. Even if you are confident that you have the right answer, you should still take the time to read each option before moving on.

General Strategies

☑ Tough Questions

If you are stumped on a problem or it appears too hard or too difficult, don't waste time. Move on! Remember though, if you can quickly check for obviously incorrect answer choices, your chances of guessing correctly are greatly improved. Before you completely give up, at least try to knock out a couple of possible answers. Eliminate what you can and then guess at the remaining answer choices before moving on.

☑ Check Your Work

Since you will probably not know every term listed and the answer to every question, it is important that you get credit for the ones that you do know. Don't miss any questions through careless mistakes. If at all possible, try to take a second to look back over your answer selection and make sure you've selected the correct answer choice and haven't made a costly careless mistake (such as marking an answer choice that you didn't mean to mark). This quick double check should more than pay for itself in caught mistakes for the time it costs.

☑ Pace Yourself

It's easy to be overwhelmed when you're looking at a page full of questions; your mind is confused and full of random thoughts, and the clock is ticking down faster than you would like. Calm down and maintain the pace that you have set for yourself. Especially as you get down to the last few minutes of the test, don't let the small numbers on the clock make you panic. As long as you are on track by monitoring your pace, you are guaranteed to have time for each question.

☑ Don't Rush

It is very easy to make errors when you are in a hurry. Maintaining a fast pace in answering questions is pointless if it makes you miss questions that you would have gotten right otherwise. Test writers like to include distracting information and wrong answers that seem right. Taking a little extra time to avoid careless mistakes can make all the difference in your test score. Find a pace that allows you to be confident in the answers that you select.

⊘ Keep Moving

Panicking will not help you pass the test, so do your best to stay calm and keep moving. Taking deep breaths and going through the answer elimination steps you practiced can help to break through a stress barrier and keep your pace.

Final Notes

The combination of a solid foundation of content knowledge and the confidence that comes from practicing your plan for applying that knowledge is the key to maximizing your performance on test day. As your foundation of content knowledge is built up and strengthened, you'll find that the strategies included in this chapter become more and more effective in helping you quickly sift through the distractions and traps of the test to isolate the correct answer.

Now that you're preparing to move forward into the test content chapters of this book, be sure to keep your goal in mind. As you read, think about how you will be able to apply this information on the test. If you've already seen sample questions for the test and you have an idea of the question format and style, try to come up with questions of your own that you can answer based on what you're reading. This will give you valuable practice applying your knowledge in the same ways you can expect to on test day.

Good luck and good studying!

Continence Care: Assessment and Care Planning

Normal Micturition and Defecation

Normal Urination

Normal urination: Kidneys produce urine, which flows through ureters into the bladder, which rests on pelvic floor muscles, extending from pubic bone to base of the spine. The bladder is enclosed in the **detrusor** muscle, creating a muscular reservoir. The bladder neck comprises the connection between the bladder and the urethra. Internal sphincter muscles and fibrous external sphincter muscles (urethral) encircle the bladder neck.

- **Phase 1: Filling/storing** is triggered by emptying the bladder. Neurotransmitters in the brain signal the detrusor muscle to relax and the bladder to expand, drawing urine from the kidney and ureters. When the bladder reaches capacity (8-16 ounces), nerves send a signal back to the brain. Voluntarily tightening the external sphincter muscles retains the urine.
- **Phase 2: Emptying** occurs when the nervous system signals the voiding reflex and spinal nerves contract the detrusor muscle and relax internal sphincter muscles, allowing urine to flow to the urethra. Relaxing external sphincter muscles allows urination.

Bladder and Urethra

The **bladder**, a muscular reservoir in the lower pelvis, provides urinary storage. The base of the bladder, an inverted triangular region known as the Trigone, contains the sensory nerves to send and receive signals and connects both ureters. The apex of the Trigone forms the bladder neck, the connection between the bladder and the urethra with the internal sphincter muscles and fibrous external sphincter muscles, which control the flow of urine from the bladder. The bladder is composed of different layers. The **mucosa** lines and protects the bladder wall and **submucosa** contains blood vessels and nerves. The **muscularis propria**, comprises the **detrusor** muscle, whose longitudinal and circular layers allow for expansion and contraction. The female urethra averages 1.5 inches long; the lining contains epithelial cells responsive to effects of estrogen. The male urethra averages 8 inches long. The proximal portion passing through the prostate, which can cause compression, is the prostatic or sphincteric urethra.

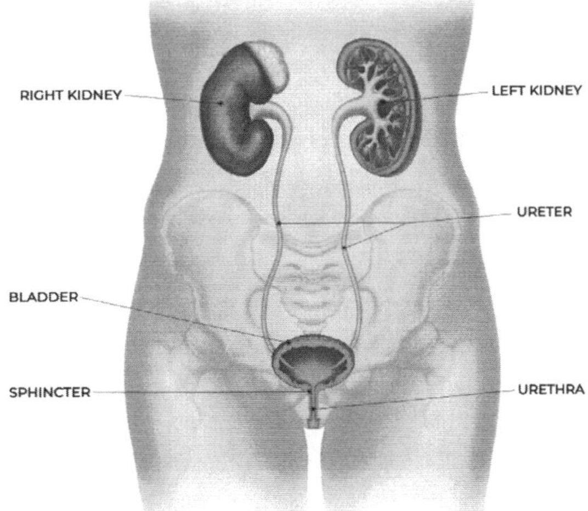

NORMAL DEFECATION

About 3-4 pints of liquid, including digested food, bile, and digestive enzymes, travel through the small intestine to the colon each day. The colon absorbs more than 90% of the fluid as the stool traverses the bowel. Undigested food takes only about 2 hours to reach the colon, but 2-5 days to reach the rectum, allowing time for reabsorption. The urge to defecate is caused when the stool travels from the sigmoid colon to the rectum. The rectosigmoid area provides storage. Eating stimulates contractions in the descending and rectosigmoid colon. The pelvic floor muscles of the rectum, including the **levator ani** and **puborectalis**, control both fecal retention and evacuation. When the rectum is distended with stool, the internal anal sphincter muscle relaxes. The external sphincter is voluntarily controlled, allowing continence. For defecation, the external anal sphincter and puborectalis muscle relax voluntarily and the pelvic floor muscles distend, propelling the stool through the anus.

Obtaining a Patient's Health History

Principles of Patient-Centered Care

Psychosocial Factors Affecting Care

Psychosocial factors affecting care include:

- **Ability to learn/perform care**: Cognitive impairment and hearing or vision deficits may interfere with the ability to learn, especially if appropriate educational materials are not available. Physical disabilities may make it difficult to patients to learn or perform some aspects of care. Language differences may result in impaired comprehension.
- **Economic implications**: Patients and families may be severely impacted if the wage earner is unable to continue to work or if they lack the resources (insurance, financial) to pay for needed care.
- **Education**: Patients may lack an adequate educational background to understand the implications of disease, to read materials, and to follow directions. Health literacy may be very low, so patients may have misconceptions about disease.
- **Mental status**: Patients often experience increased stress associated with illness, and this may interfere with functioning. Mental impairment may impact ability to participate in care. Additionally, depression is common, especially with chronic illness, and may cause patients to withdraw or fail to comply with treatment.

Cultural Beliefs

Cultural beliefs may influence patients' understanding of disease, emotional response, and acceptance of treatment. It's important to ask patients about cultural preferences, to avoid making assumptions, and to respect patients' beliefs. Issues to consider include:

- **Shame**: Some may believe that wounds or drainage, especially fecal, bring shame or uncleanliness. They may have stigma about body image. Education and support are especially important to help overcome shame.
- **Traditional treatments**: Some may rely on healers or nonstandard treatments, such as poultices and herbal medications. As much as possible, these approaches should be included in the plan of care.
- **Family roles**: Decision-making may be made by someone other than the patient, such as by the eldest member of the family or the male head of the family. Showing respect for this tradition is essential for cooperation.
- **Gender**: Some cultures may resist treatment of a patient by the opposite gender. It's important to always ask permission before caring for or touching a patient.
- **Pain**: Some cultures may express pain more openly than others or may not understand the 0-10 scale often used for assessment, so the nurse should use various methods of assessment and make careful observations.

Informed Consent

The **Patient Self Determination Act** (1991) confirms the right for patients to give informed consent. Patients or family must provide informed consent for all treatment the patient receives. This includes a thorough explanation of all procedures and treatment and associated risks. Patients/family should be apprised of all options and allowed input on the type of treatments. Patients/family should be apprised of all reasonable risks and any complications that might be life threatening or increase morbidity. The American Medical Association has established guidelines for informed consent:

- Explanation of diagnosis
- Nature and reason for treatment or procedure
- Risks and benefits
- Alternative options (regardless of cost or insurance coverage)
- Risks and benefits of alternative options
- Risks and benefits of not having a treatment or procedure
- Providing informed consent is a requirement of all states

Health Literacy

Health literacy is the ability to obtain, understand, and consent to medical care, making informed healthcare decisions and must be considered when developing activities. Health literacy includes:

- Reading with comprehension, applying reason to context.
- Understanding graphs and other visual representations of information.
- Using the computer to obtain information.
- Understanding the results of laboratory/radiographic studies.
- Understanding and using basic mathematical computations.
- Articulating concerns and questions.
- Understanding basic anatomy and physiology.
- Having basic knowledge of disease.
- Understanding preventive health measures.
- Knowing how to access health care and health information.

Health literacy may be impacted by a number of factors, including lack of adequate education (low reading level), illiteracy, dementia, and learning disabilities. Those most vulnerable include the elderly, ethnic minorities, immigrants, and those with low income and/or chronic medical or physical health problems. The nurse must evaluate the patient/caregiver to determine their level of health literacy and gear education to that level.

Supporting Patient and Caregiver Goals

Preventive goals: Measures to prevent disease/disability or prevent deterioration or complications of existing disorder. May include screening (BP, Pap smear, mammograms, blood glucose), disease education, fall prevention, smoking cessation, substance abuse rehabilitation, vaccinations, nutritional counseling, and exercise.

Maintenance goals: Measures to control existing disorder in order to maintain status. May include therapy (OT, PT, ST), education, ongoing lifestyle changes, supervision, ongoing assessment, medications, blood glucose management, and treatment. Maintenance therapy may follow primary therapy for some diseases, such as cancer, in order to maintain status.

Curative goals: Measures intended to cure disease rather than simply to alleviate symptoms or pain. May include medications, casting (as for broken limbs), radiotherapy, dialysis, transfusions, chemotherapy, physical therapy, rehabilitation therapy, and surgical interventions. Note: Curative treatments are also sometimes used for palliation but without intent to cure.

Access to Care

A number of factors may affect **access to care**:

- **Proximity to medical services**: Some geographic areas have more medical services than others. For example, some rural areas lack both hospitals and physicians. Cutting edge treatments may be unavailable in some areas.
- **Socioeconomic status**: Lack of insurance or money to pay for medical services prevents many people from seeking medical care or complying with treatments. Many cannot afford to pay for prescription drugs or supplies.
- **Language differences**: Non-English speakers may not be able to communicate needs or to understand information, such as the treatment plan.
- **Health literacy**: Some may have little knowledge and understanding of anatomy, physiology, disease, and medical treatments.
- **Disability status**: Disabilities may have a profound effect of access to care or very little, depending on the type of disability and the resources available, but some disabilities impair mobility and the ability to access care.
- **Transportation**: Private and public transportation may be unavailable or the cost prohibitive.
- **Race and ethnicity**: Inequalities faced by minority populations often extend to medical services. Many live in poor neighborhoods that provide little access to medical services.

Interview Process

The nurse should review previous medical records and have a clear idea of the purpose of the **interview** and should outline questions. If possible, the patient should be interviewed alone or should be asked if he/she wants family members present. Both verbal and nonverbal responses should be observed during an interview. Important factors include:

- **Initial introductions**: Make introductions by name and explain roles and the purpose of the interview, asking how the patient wishes to be addressed and avoiding using familiar terms, such as "dear," which may be considered condescending. Stress the confidential nature of the interview and explain who will receive the information.
- **Interview structure**: The interview may be somewhat unstructured, guided by patient responses, or may be very structured with the nurse asking a list of questions, but the nurse must remain flexible while still guiding the discussion in order to accommodate different communication styles.
- **Appearance**: The nurse should be professionally dressed and wearing a clear nametag. The patient's appearance should be observed non-judgmentally for clothes (loose/tight clothes may indicate weight change), cleanliness (dirty clothes/skin/hair may indicate cognitive or physical impairment or poverty), and demeanor (calm, fidgeting, nervous).

Environmental Assessment

Areas in Home

Environmental assessments are very helpful when developing a care plan to provide for care and safety. Rooms should be assessed according to their function:

- **Entryway** should be free of obstacles and surfaces even. Handrails and/or ramps may be needed for those who are unsteady or wheelchair bound.
- **Stairs/steps** should have handrails, non-skid surfaces, and contrast markings for each step.
- **Living area** should be comfortable and furniture arranged for convenience. Chairs should be firm enough for people to stand from easily.
- **Bedrooms** should have a night light and phone near the bed. Bed should be positioned close to the nearest bathroom if possible and at the appropriate height for easy access and appropriate firmness.
- **Bathrooms** might need grab bars, hand-held shower, and elevated toilet seat, tub seat.
- **Kitchen** may need items moved for convenient access as well as a sturdy step stool. Unsafe equipment/tools should be removed.

General Elements

Some elements of environmental assessment are not specific to rooms in the house but are general needs that must be met in order for people, especially the elderly or disabled, to remain safe:

- **Environmental hazards** such as piles of papers or junk on the floors, loose carpet or rugs, and cluttered pathways can cause falls and must be cleared, organized, or repaired.
- **Lighting** should be adequate enough for reading in all rooms and stairways.
- **Heat and air conditioning** must be adequate. The young and the elderly are especially susceptible to heat and cold injury.
- **Sanitation** should ensure that health hazards do not exist, such as from rotting food or infestations of cockroaches or rodents.
- **Animals** should be cared for adequately with access to food, water, toileting, and routine veterinary care.
- **Smoke/chemicals** in the environment may pose a hazard, such as exposure to cigarette smoking or cleaning materials.

Assessing Current and Historical Environmental Factors

Environmental factors should be assessed within the actual environment if at all possible. If not, careful questioning and drawing of diagrams and approximate floor plans with the patient—or asking the patient to do drawings—can be useful, especially when showing the patient needed modifications. Family members may also assist with the assessment, providing useful information. Some patients, especially the elderly, may be reluctant to admit that the home is cluttered or that they are unable to maintain the home environment in a sanitary condition. Brochures and handouts about home safety and assistive devices should be provided to the patient as well as contact names and numbers for equipment needed in the home. A checklist should be compiled of all necessary changes or additions, with specific details, such as "Install 18-inch grab bar across from toilet." In some cases, a social worker or occupational therapist should visit the patient.

Assessing Current and Historical Functional Abilities

Functional abilities should be assessed in an active manner, with the person demonstrating the ability to sit, stand, get on and off of the toilet, walk, bend down, remove clothing and then put it on again, listen, read, and answer questions. Ideally, this should be in the home environment, but careful questioning about distances and type of facilities in the home environment can help with approximating the type of activities required. The person can walk up and down a hallway, for example, to approximate walking from the car to the front door. A careful history of functional ability can pinpoint when and if changes occurred. Again, specific questioning guides people, "When did you begin to use a cane?" "How old were you when you stopped using the tub?" "What is the biggest problem with caring for yourself?" or "When did you have a hysterectomy/prostatectomy, and how has that changed your life?"

Considering Risk Factors for Incontinence

Functional Status Assessment

Functional status assessment concerns the ability to do self-care, self-maintenance, and engage in physical activities, but other factors may prevent those who should be able to function well from doing so:

- **Psychological function** assesses anxiety, worry, grief, and depression. Those with depression may be at increased risk of physical disability or may neglect self-care.
- **Social function** assesses support from family or friends, the need for a caregiver, financial resources, mistreatment or abuse, the ability to drive, and the presence of advance directives.
- **Sensory function** assesses presence of cataracts, glaucoma, myopia, presbyopia, astigmatism, macular degeneration, or eye disorders that make it difficult for people to read medication labels or do self-care. The need for audio materials or enlarged print should be assessed. Hearing is evaluated in both ears for hearing deficits and high and low frequency hearing loss as well as waxy buildup in the ear canals.

Functional status relates to the ability of people, especially the elderly, to perform social roles free of limitations or disabilities. Assessment should include basic activities of daily living:

- **Toileting** assesses the ability to adequately control urination and fecal evacuation, noting dysuria, constipation, diarrhea, the presence and degree of incontinence, and the use of protective materials.
- **Mobility** assesses the ability to transfer from bed to chair, to walk, to toilet, and to maintain balance, noting recent falls or the need for assistive devices.
- **Hygiene** assesses the ability to bathe, brush teeth, dress, and maintain basic standards of cleanliness both for the person and the environment.
- **Mental** status assesses thinking, understanding, and memory because, by age 90, about 50% of people have some dementia.
- **Nutrition** assesses basic dietary knowledge, the ability to prepare or obtain food, and adequate food and fluid intake.

Pharmacological and Surgical History

Pharmacological history should include a complete list of all current and past medications, including over the counter or herbal medications, and people questioned about dosage to determine if they are taking medications and treatments properly. As with medical history, specific questions should be asked, "Have you taken hormone replacement therapy, such as estrogen?" rather than "What medicines have you taken?" People should also be asked specifically whether they have had chemotherapy, when, and for what?

Surgical history should include specific questions about surgical procedures rather than "Have you ever had any surgeries" because people may forget or omit surgeries in the distant past. It may be helpful to also ask people if they have any surgical scars as that may elicit more information. Men should be asked specifically if they have had a prostatectomy or vasectomy and women if they have had a hysterectomy or other gynecological or urological surgical repair.

Medical History

Medical history should be assessed carefully with specific questions related to each body system rather than general questions, such as "Have you ever had a major illness?" Additionally, people should be asked if they have had any tumors, cancers, or lumps and ever had or been treated for psychological problems, such as anxiety, depression, and alcohol or drug abuse. As well as specific disorders, people should be questioned about common symptoms such as dizziness, tingling, headaches, incontinence, or weakness. Detailed questions about genitourinary history should include sexual issues, such as ejaculatory or impotence problems, painful intercourse, menstrual cycles or dysmenorrhea, menopause, and any urinary problems. A medical assessment should include radiation therapy (especially to the pelvic area), the need for or use of assistive devices, and any history of allergic reactions. General information about people's background, such as marital status, number of children, and educational status can help to formulate a care plan.

Assessing Cognitive Abilities

Assessment of cognitive abilities may only be officially conducted with permission of the patient or a legal representative or it can be considered an assault, so obtaining permission before beginning the assessment or documenting emergency evaluation is necessary. A medical and social history should be done before assessing cognitive abilities. During the assessment, appearance, eye contact, and affect should be documented.

The **Mini-Mental State Exam** is an assessment tool that provides a quantitative measure of cognitive status of adults. It can be used for initial assessment, to follow the patient's changes over time, and to evaluate the effectiveness of treatment. The test packet includes detachable sheets with stimuli for tasks related to comprehension, reading, writing, and drawing. The assessment tests speech, thought processes and content, hallucinations or abnormal thoughts, orientation to date, time, and place, concentration, ability to read and write, and abstract reasoning through a variety of tasks and questions.

Lifestyle Assessment

Lifestyle issues may change from one period of life to another, so specifically asking about current and past habits as well as changes that might have taken place is important. A non-judgmental attitude, assuring people that these questions can help to provide the best care to them, helps people be more forthcoming when providing this information.

- **Drug habits** should be assessed with specific questions about common drugs, such as marijuana, cocaine, crack, and heroin, but also prescription drugs, such as Vicodin or valium, including questions about length of use and last or current use of drugs and whether the people had treatment for addiction.
- **Alcohol intake** should be assessed with specific questions about how much and when people drink. "What time during the day do you take your first drink?" "How many drinks do you have in a normal day?" "Describe one typical drink." It's important also to ask if drinking has ever caused problems in their lives or if they have ever had treatment or attended a program to stop drinking.
- **Bowel habits** should include frequency and appearance of stools, history of constipation, diarrhea, painful evacuation, bloody stools, or incontinence.
- **Bladder habits** should include frequency of urination and appearance of urine, history of nocturia, hematuria, dysuria, and any incontinence. Men should be questioned about difficulty initiating flow or emptying bladder.
- **Diet** should include a typical day's menu, including number of meals and meal times. People should be asked specifically if they have been on any special diets, for weight loss or other health reasons. Vegetarians or vegans should be questioned about protein in their diets. Food allergies should be noted as well.
- **Hydration** should include amount and types of fluids (water and others), with specific questions, such as "What do you drink with breakfast?"
- **Smoking** assessment should include when the people first started smoking, what they smoke, and how much: "How many cigarettes do you smoke in one day?" and "How soon after you wake up do you have your first cigarette?" Assessment should include length of time people smoked, when they quit, attempts to quit, and questions about anyone living in the home or close associates who smoke.
- **Obesity** questions should avoid words like "fat" and "obese," but focus on specifics, such as "How long have you been at your current weight?" "How much did you weigh at age 20?" "How much has your weight fluctuated?" "Are you unhappy with your weight" and "Have you tried exercise or weight loss programs?"
- **Exercise** assessment should include what type of exercise people do, how often, and how long, such as "Where did you walk yesterday?" "How long did you walk?" and "What equipment do you use at the gym?"

SEXUAL HISTORY

Sexual history is an important part of any assessment for all ages and may elicit information that is helpful in diagnosing urinary or fecal incontinence. Multiple partners, certain sexual practices, or trauma may increase the risk of developing problems that can lead to urinary or fecal incontinence.

- Is the person sexually active? If so, how many partners? Are partners of the same sex, opposite sex, or both sexes?
- Is there a history of sexually transmitted diseases, such as chlamydia and gonorrhea?
- Does the person use birth control methods? What type?
- Is sexual activity painful or uncomfortable? Is there leakage of urine during sex?
- Is the woman post-menopause? If so, are there changes in sexual comfort, or urinary or fecal disorders?
- Are there erectile problems or difficulty with urination indicating an enlarged prostate?
- Is there history of sexual trauma, such as sexual abuse or surgical procedures?

VOIDING AND BOWEL DYSFUNCTION SPECIFIC TO PEDIATRIC POPULATION

ENURESIS

Enuresis is repeated involuntary urinary incontinence in children old enough to have bladder control, usually about 5-6 years old. Diabetes and other disorders should be ruled out although 95% are not associated with structural or neurological disorders. There are three types:

- **Primary**: The child has never been dry at night, and incontinence is associated with delay in maturation and small functional bladder rather than stress or psychiatric disorders.
- **Intermittent**: The child stays dry part of the time with episodes of incontinence at night.
- **Secondary**: The child has had long periods (6-12 months) staying dry and then is incontinent because of infection, stress, or sleep disorder.

Treatment includes:

- Laboratory assessment and examination to rule out primary causes.
- Fluid restriction.
- Bladder training.
- Enuresis alarms.
- Imipramine (tricyclic antidepressant) is used with many children but require close monitoring.
- Desmopressin nasal spray may be used for short-term control.
- Support and acceptance.

POSTERIOR URETHRAL VALVES

Posterior urethral valves (PUV) are a urethral abnormality in males where urethral valves have narrow slit-like openings that impede urinary flow and allow reverse flow, damaging urinary organs, which swell and become engorged with urine. Thirty percent with PUV will develop long-term kidney failure. **Symptoms** vary depending upon severity:

- **Dysuria**: Pain, weak stream, frequency.
- Hematuria. Urinary retention. Incontinence. Enlarged bladder palpable as abdominal mass. Urinary infection (most common symptom after 1 year of age). Sepsis, metabolic acidosis, and azotemia (increased blood levels of urea and other nitrogenous compounds) may develop.

Diagnosis consists of:

- Fetal ultrasound.
- Voiding cystourethrogram (VCUG): Evaluate extent of valvular abnormality and other urinary defects.
- Endoscopy: Examine inside of urinary tract/take tissue samples. Blood tests: Assess kidney function and electrolytes.

Treatment includes:

- Supportive care, antibiotics, electrolytes, Foley catheter.
- Urinary diversion: Usually closed after valve repair.
- Endoscopic ablation/resection: Examine obstruction and remove valve leaflets.

VESICOURETERAL REFLUX

Vesicoureteral reflux is an abnormality where urine flows from the bladder back up the ureter. Reflux is graded on a scale of 1-5, depending upon the degree of dilation of the ureter and renal pelvis.

- **Primary**: Congenital defect with impaired valve where ureter opens to bladder. The ureter may be too short so the valve doesn't close properly.
- **Secondary**: Caused by infection or other cause of obstruction.

Symptoms of urinary tract infection are most common:

- **Neonates**: Fever, irritability, lethargy, emesis.
- **Older infants, children**: Abdominal pain, emesis, diarrhea, fever, dysuria with enuresis, frequency, urgency, cloudy/foul urine.
- **Late symptoms**: Hypertension, dysuria with difficulty urinating, proteinuria, chronic renal insufficiency.

Diagnosis is by:

- **Ultrasound**: Evaluate appearance of urinary system.
- **Voiding cystourethrogram (VCUG)**: Identify reflux (after infection has cleared).
- **Intravenous pyelogram**: Reveal obstructions.
- **Nuclear scans**: Show urinary functioning
- **Cystoscopy**: View bladder interior.

Treatment includes:

- **Antibiotics**: For infection.
- **Surgical repair/reconstruction**: Usually involves severing ureter from bladder and reattaching at a different angle to prevent reflux.

Epispadias and Hypospadias

Epispadias is a condition in which the urethral orifice is in an abnormal position with a widened pubic bone. In boys, the urethra may open on the top (dorsum), the sides, or the complete length of the penis. In girls, the urethra, with a urethral cleft along its length, usually bifurcates the clitoris and labia but may be in the abdomen. Boys may have a short, wide penis with abnormal chordee (curvature). Epispadias is 3-5 times more common in males than females. **Hypospadias**, which occurs only in males, is a condition in which the urethral orifice opens onto the ventral surface of the penis.

Diagnosis is by physical exam and endoscopy to evaluate bladder neck and external sphincter. Intravenous pyelogram evaluates the urinary tract.

Symptoms for both conditions include urinary incontinence, infections, and reflux nephropathy (backward flow of urine to kidneys). **Treatment** is surgical repair to lengthen the urethra (and penis, in males) and reconstruct the bladder neck. Multiple surgical procedures may be required for both males and females. Urinary diversion may be necessary if incontinence cannot be corrected.

Hirschsprung Disease

Hirschsprung's disease **(congenital aganglionic megacolon)** is failure of **ganglion nerve cells** to migrate to part of the bowel, usually the distal colon, so that part of the bowel lacks enervation and peristalsis, causing stool to accumulate, leading to **distention** and **megacolon**. There is a genetic predisposition to the disease that affects more males than females and is associated with trisomy 21 (Down syndrome).

Symptoms include:

- Failure to pass meconium in 24 to 48 hours
- Poor feeding
- Bilious vomitus
- Abdominal distension

Delayed diagnosis includes:

- Chronic constipation
- Failure to thrive
- Periods of diarrhea and vomiting
- With infection—severe prostration, watery diarrhea, fever, and hypotension

Treatment includes:

- Resection aganglionic section and perform colorectal anastomosis.
- There are a number of procedures, but recently, minimally invasive laparoscopic or transanal approaches have proven successful.

Ureteropelvic Junction Obstruction

Ureteropelvic junction obstruction (UPJ) is congenital obstruction at the point where the ureter connects to the renal pelvis, unilaterally or bilaterally, causing inadequate urinary flow and hydronephrosis. Some children improve markedly within the first 18 months, but others require surgery. **Symptoms** include:

- Urinary tract infections. Abdominal or flank pain
- Palpable mass from hydronephrosis. Vomiting.

Diagnosis is based on:

- **Fetal ultrasound**: in utero diagnosis.
- **Renal ultrasound**: To show dilation of renal pelvis.
- **Intravenous pyelogram (IVP)**: To identify obstruction.
- **Renal isotope scan**: To evaluate and measure kidney function.

Treatment includes:

- **Fetal urinary diversion**: Remains controversial.
- **Pyeloplasty**: Open surgical procedure where ureteropelvic junction is excised and ureter reattached to renal pelvis with wide junction, allowing adequate drainage.
- **Laparoscopic pyeloplasty**: Through abdominal wall and abdominal cavity with internal excision of ureteropelvic junction.
- **Insertion of wire through ureter**: To cut ureteropelvic junction from inside with a ureteral drain left in place for a few weeks.

Malrotation and Volvulus

Malrotation is a congenital defect in which the intestines are attached to the back of the abdominal wall by one single attachment rather than a broad band of attachments across the abdomen, essentially suspending the bowels so that they can easily twist, resulting in a **volvulus** (twisted bowel), cutting off blood supply. It may untwist but can lead to bowel infraction. Some children with malrotation have no symptoms, but most develop **symptoms** by one year:

- Cycles of cramping pain about every 15-30 minutes that cause the child to cry and pull knees to chest.
- Distended painful abdomen, diarrhea, bloody stools, or no stools.
- Vomiting (occurring soon after crying begins usually indicates small intestine obstruction; later vomiting usually indicated large intestine blockage).
- Tachycardia and tachypnea.
- Decreased urinary output.
- Fever.

Treatment includes surgical repair (Ladd procedure), which is indicated immediately if there is volvulus and most malrotations require surgical repair even with less severe symptoms.

Urinary Incontinence

Causes of Urinary Incontinence

The following are common causes of urinary incontinence:

- **Pregnancy/childbirth**: Childbirth weakens the pelvic floor muscles and those of the urethral sphincter. Nerve damage and bladder prolapse can also occur, further contributing to incontinence.
- **Post-menopausal changes**: Loss of estrogen causes bladder and urethral tissues to weaken.
- **Hysterectomy**: The muscles and nerves in the urinary tract may be damaged by the procedure because the urinary tract is adjacent to the uterus.
- **Interstitial cystitis**: The inflammation sometimes causes incontinence.
- **Prostate enlargement**: Constriction of the urethra as the prostate enlarges can lead to urgency or overflow incontinence.
- **Prostate cancer**: May be caused directly by the cancer or may be a response to radiation or surgical removal of prostate.
- **Bladder cancer**: Dysuria and incontinence are common symptoms.
- **Neurological deficits**: Congenital or acquired neurological damage from injury or disease can result in inability to control urination.
- **Urinary tract obstruction**: An obstruction anywhere in the urinary tract can cause overflow incontinence.

Menopause and Urinary or Fecal Incontinence

Menopause is a major cause of urinary incontinence with about 40% of post-menopausal women developing the disorder to some degree. Estrogen maintains the lining of the bladder and the urethra and stimulates the flow of blood to the pelvic area. As levels of estrogen begin to drop with menopause, the muscles are less well-nourished and the lining of the bladder and urethra may become dry and irritated. The sphincter muscles may lose tone as well. Until recent years, many women took hormone replacement therapy (HRT), believing this protected them from the effects of aging, but subsequent studies have shown that HRT, in fact, increased the risk of urinary incontinence and did not have the same protective effect as natural estrogen, posing yet another risk factor. In addition to the loss of natural estrogen, weight gain after menopause increases the stress on the bladder and the supporting muscles, adding to the risk of urinary incontinence.

Management of Transient Urinary Incontinence

Transient urinary incontinence is a reversible or temporary condition caused by a number of clinical conditions. Management, therefore, is concerned with first identifying the cause, and then treating it.

- **Impaction** usually is related to chronic constipation. Bowel training and dietary modifications, including increased fiber in diet, should be instigated.
- **Dementia** may be from a disease, such as Alzheimer's, surgery, or medications. If related to Alzheimer's medications, such as Aricept, Exelon, or Namenda, may help. Scheduled toileting and absorbent pads or briefs may be necessary.
- **Urinary tract infections** require antibiotics and adequate fluid intake.
- **Vaginitis, urethritis** may respond to topical estrogen.
- **Chronic diseases** should be controlled adequately with medications and treatments as needed.

- **Chronic pain** should be assessed and a plan for pain control put in place.
- **Decreased mobility** may require assistive devices, such as elevated toilet seats, safety bars, urinals, commode chairs.
- **Medications** may need to be changed.

TRANSIENT CAUSES OF URINARY INCONTINENCE

CLINICAL CONDITIONS

Transient causes of urinary incontinence are reversible or temporary. A number of clinical conditions can affect the urinary system.

- **Impaction** may distend the rectum and anus, causing pressure on bladder neck, obstructing urinary flow, resulting in overflow incontinence.
- **Dementia** may result from illness, such as stroke, as well as surgery or medications. People may lose awareness of need to urinate or use of toilet.
- **Urinary tract infections** can cause frequency and urge incontinence.
- **Vaginitis, urethritis** with atrophic muscle changes can cause incontinence.
- **Yeast infections**, such as *Candida albicans,* result in irritation about the vagina, vulva, and urethra, resulting in burning, frequency, and urge incontinence.
- **Chronic illnesses** (diabetes mellitus or other disorders associated with polyuria and conditions with edema, such as heart failure) may cause urge incontinence.
- **Chronic pain** results in inattention to toileting needs.
- **Decreased mobility** prevents response to urge to urinate.

PSYCHOLOGICAL CONDITIONS, LIFESTYLE ISSUES, AND GENDER-SPECIFIC DISORDERS

Psychological conditions, such as severe depression, can impair the ability of a person to take care of basic needs, such as toileting.

Lifestyle issues that can cause incontinence by putting pressure on the bladder and pelvic floor muscles include obesity that weakens pelvic floor muscles, poor hygiene that causes chronic urinary tract infections, poor bowel habits that cause chronic straining for a bowel movement, and smoking, resulting in chronic cough that causes stress incontinence.

Gender-specific disorders obstruction, urinary retention, and/or incontinence. In males, an enlarged prostate may compress the urethra, causing an obstruction that results in urinary retention and overflow incontinence. Prostatectomy, on the other hand, can cause damage that result in stress incontinence. In females, a history of trauma related to childbirth, especially with multiparity, can cause stress incontinence. Pelvic radiation for both men and women can result in radiation damage to tissue that can affect bladder function.

MEDICATIONS

Medications may contribute to urinary incontinence:

- **Diuretics**, such as furosemide, hydrochlorothiazide, and caffeine can cause polyuria.
- **Sedative and hypnotics**, such as benzodiazepines and alcohol can cause confusion and depress inhibition to urinate.
- **Antihypertensives**, such as prazosin, terazosin, doxazosin, and methyldopa can cause relaxation of the urethral sphincter.
- **Narcotics**, such as morphine sulfate or meperidine can cause confusion and decrease bladder contractions, causing retention.

- **Anti-seizures**, such as thioridazine, chlorpromazine, haloperidol, and clozapine may cause enuresis because of alpha-blocker effect.
- **Anti-anxiety/muscle relaxants**, such as those of the benzodiazepine class—diazepam, alprazolam, and clonazepam--can weaken the external urethral sphincter.
- **Antidepressants/antipsychotics**, such as amitriptyline, nortriptyline and other tricyclics can decrease bladder contractions, causing retention.
- **Antihistamines**, such as chlorpheniramine and diphenhydramine, can cause decreased bladder contractions with retention.
- **Anti-Parkinson agents** cause decreased bladder contractions with retention.
- Polypharmacy can cause interactions leading to incontinence.

Dietary Factors

Dietary factors can result in incontinence:

- **Caffeine** occurs naturally in coffee beans, tealeaves, and cocoa beans. Caffeine is added to many soft drinks. It is in chocolate drinks and candy. Additionally, it is also an additive in many drugs, such as Excedrin, Anacin, Darvon compounds, and Fiorinal. Caffeine can increase detrusor muscle contractions, causing increased pressure that can result in urinary urgency and frequency.
- **Artificial sweeteners** (aspartame, NutraSweet, and saccharine) are bladder irritants.
- **Citrus foods**, such as orange juice and cranberry juice are highly acidic and irritate the lining of the bladder and can worsen overactive bladder and urge incontinence.
- **Spicy foods**, such as Mexican or Chinese food, horseradish, and chili peppers irritate the bladder lining, similar to citrus foods.
- **Fluid intake** in excess of 32-48 ounces per day can worsen both stress and urge incontinence. Alcohol, especially, acts as a diuretic and acts directly on the bladder.

Reversible Causes of Incontinence

Reversible causes of incontinence include:

- **Delirium** is an acute sudden change in consciousness, characterized by reduced ability to focus or sustain attention, language and memory disturbance, disorientation, confusion, audiovisual hallucinations, sleep disturbance, incontinence, and psychomotor activity disorder. Delirium differs from disorders with similar symptoms in that delirium is fluctuating. Delirium occurs in 10-40% of hospitalized older adults and about 80% of patients who are terminally ill.
- **Fecal impaction** occurs when the hard stool moves into the rectum and becomes a large, dense, immovable mass that cannot be evacuated even with straining, usually as a result of chronic constipation. In addition to abdominal cramps and distention, the person may feel intense rectal pressure and pain accompanied by a sense of urgency to defecate. Nausea and vomiting may also occur. Hemorrhoids will often become engorged. Fecal incontinence, with liquid stool leaking about the impaction, is common.
- **Infection**, such as urinary tract infection or vaginal infection, may result in urinary incontinence, which usually clears once the infection is effectively treated.

Risk Factors for Urinary Incontinence

The following are risk factors for urinary incontinence:

- **Age**: Bladder and sphincter muscles loosen with age, so the older a person is, the more likely to have some type of urinary incontinence, stress or chronic.
- **Contributing diseases**: Kidney diseases, among others, may make an individual prone to develop urinary incontinence if the conditions are not well controlled.
- **Obesity**: Being overweight increases pressure on the bladder and the surrounding muscles, weakening them and causing stress incontinence. This is especially true for women.
- **Sex**: Women are more likely to suffer incontinence than men because of childbirth and menopausal changes. Also, the genitourinary anatomy of women with the vagina/bladder/urethra/rectum adjacent contributes to the danger of injury to the urinary system.
- **Smoking**: The chronic cough that many smokers develop can cause stress incontinence or can aggravate stress incontinence that is already present.
- **Sports**: High impact sports with vigorous activity, such as running, can put strong pressure on the bladder during those activities.

Urinary Infections

Urinary infections can occur anywhere within the urinary tract. Cystitis, a bladder infection, is very common, especially in women because the urethra is very short and bacteria from the anal area can easily migrate to the bladder. The most common cause is the bacteria *E. coli*, which is part of the natural flora of the intestine. Untreated cystitis can result in the infection spreading to the kidneys. Urinary infections are also common in people who are elderly and dehydrated, such as those in nursing homes, and those with diabetes. Chronic bacteriuria may develop in older females, especially those with indwelling Foley catheters. *Chlamydia* and *Mycoplasma* may also cause urethral urinary infections in both males and females and is sexually transmitted. Urinary infection can cause swelling and inflammation of the mucosa and painful bladder spasms, often resulting in urinary incontinence, especially urge incontinence, in which the urge to urinate is immediately followed by involuntary urination.

Pelvic Organ Prolapse

Pelvic organ prolapse occurs when pelvic floor muscles weaken from age, trauma, or other causes and cannot support the pelvic organs, causing them to prolapse or protrude, primarily through the vaginal wall. Some types of prolapse are frequently associated with urinary incontinence.

- **Cystoceles** often result in urinary incontinence, especially during sexual intercourse when there is pressure exerted against the prolapsing bladder. Stress incontinence is also common.
- **Urethroceles** are also implicated in urinary incontinence because of impairment of function resulting from the prolapse.
- **Uterine prolapse**, depending upon the severity, may apply pressure on the bladder and urethra, preventing complete emptying of the bladder and resulting in frequent urinary tract infections with urinary frequency, urgency, and incontinence.
- **Rectoceles** are most often associated with fecal incontinence but some people may have both urinary and fecal incontinence.
- **Enteroceles** are only rarely associated with urinary incontinence usually when the enterocele is quite large.

Predisposing Factors

There are a number of different factors that contribute to pelvic organ prolapse:

- **Trauma** related to pregnancy and childbirth is the primary cause of pelvic organ prolapse because labor and birth causes stress on the pelvic muscles and ligaments, especially if forceps are used to facilitate vaginal delivery or an episiotomy is performed.
- **Previous pelvic surgery**, especially hysterectomy or bladder repair, may damage nerves and tissues, increasing risk for prolapse.
- **Obesity** exerts pressure on the pelvic floor muscles.
- **Chronic cough/strain**, as may occur with chronic obstructive pulmonary disease or long-term smoking, may weaken the pelvic structures over prolonged periods of time.
- **Heavy lifting** can cause damage to pelvic muscles.
- **Spinal cord damage** whether congenital or acquired may cause paralysis or atrophy of the pelvic muscles, thereby weakening the support.

Fistula

Fistulas are abnormal tunnel-like openings usually between 2 organs, or from an organ to the surface of the skin, often originating from an abscess. Fistulas involving the anus, rectum, or vagina and the perineal tissue can result in damage to intestinal and pelvic floor muscles, nerves, and sphincters.

- **Vesicovaginal** and **ureterovaginal** fistulas are common complications of female pelvic surgery, especially after a hysterectomy. The urinary incontinence that develops from these types of fistulas resembles symptoms of stress incontinence, but develops soon after surgery. Leakage occurring both during the day and night is also suggestive of vesicovaginal fistula. Surgical repair of the fistulas may, in itself, cause damage to nerves or muscles, resulting in persistent urinary incontinence.
- **Vesicouterine fistulas** are most commonly related to low segment Cesarean sections and may present with urinary incontinence. Urinary incontinence after gynecological surgery is often indication of fistula formation and should prompt urological examination.

Prostate Disease

Prostate disease is an abnormal condition of the male reproductive gland that surrounds the urethra, just below the level of the bladder.

- **Benign prostatic hypertrophy/hyperplasia** usually does not develop until after age 40 but results from the second growth phase that begins at about age 25. The prostate may slowly enlarge, but the tissue encapsulating it restrains outward growth, so the gland compresses the urethra. The bladder wall also goes through changes, becoming thicker and irritated, so that it begins to spasm, causing frequent urinations. The bladder muscle eventually weakens and the bladder fails to empty completely. People may suffer urgency, dribbling, frequency, nocturia, and urge incontinence.
- **Prostate cancer**, depending on lesion size and location, may cause similar symptoms, and resulting surgical removal or external beam radiation may result in nerve and muscle damage causing loss or compromise of bladder control although nerve-sparing techniques may minimize these complications.

CANCER

Cancer of the pelvic organs may compromise the urinary tract. Invasive cancer of the bladder may result in cystectomy and urinary diversion or bladder reconstruction, using segments of the small or large intestine to create a urinary reservoir. One complication of this type of surgery is occasional or chronic urinary incontinence. Prostate, cervical, rectal, and urethral cancers can also cause urinary incontinence because of nerve or muscle damage. Cancers outside of the pelvis may also be implicated. Lung or esophageal cancer that causes chronic cough may result in persistent stress incontinence because of weakening of pelvic floor muscles. Breast cancer may result in hormonal changes in the vaginal and urethral mucosa that cause drying and prevent the urethral sphincter from closing tightly. Treatments for cancer may also cause urinary incontinence. Radiation to the pelvic area may cause irritation of the bladder and urge incontinence. High doses of chemotherapy may cause chronic bladder irritation.

PELVIC PAIN SYNDROME

Pelvic pain syndrome is characterized by persistent or recurrent episodes of pelvic pain that is associated with urinary, sexual, bowel, or gynecological dysfunction despite lack of evident infection or other pathology and is continuous or recurrent for 6 months or more. The distribution and intensity of pain can vary considerably from one individual to another and may involve many different organs and structures. The particular aspects of pelvic pain syndrome that relate to urinary incontinence are **bladder pain syndrome, urethral pain syndrome, prostate pain syndrome, penile pain syndrome, and scrotal pain syndrome.** Prostate pain in males is often associated with a nonspecific prostatitis and may be experienced as pain at the base of the penis and around the anus. All of these manifestations may present with urological disorders, including pain on urination, failure to empty the bladder because of pain, and urinary overflow resulting in urinary incontinence.

TRAUMA

Trauma to the urinary system may involve both blunt and penetrating injuries. Blunt trauma to the abdomen may result in kidney, bladder, or ureteral damage as well as damage to the external genitalia. Vaginal injuries not related to childbirth, such as from sexual abuse or other penetrating injuries, have coexisting urological injuries in about 30% of cases. People sustaining back or flank penetrating wounds and pelvic trauma are at risk for damage to the urinary system. Injury to the bladder during automobile accidents is common because of the impact of the seat back to the lower abdomen. If the damage is severe, there may be a tear through the wall of the bladder and the vagina, causing urine to leak through the vagina. Gunshot wounds and stab injuries may cause extensive damage. Almost all trauma to the urinary system initially presents with hematuria, but untreated may develop into abscesses and fistulas and various other urinary tract symptoms, including urinary incontinence.

NEUROMUSCULAR CONDITIONS

Neuromuscular conditions include a wide range of neurodegenerative disorders, traumatic nerve injuries, toxic metabolic disorders of the peripheral nerves and muscles, and autoimmune neuromuscular disorders, many causing damage to muscles and nerves affecting urinary function, including the following:

- **Parkinson disease** is a chronic progressive neurodegenerative disease that affects both voluntary and involuntary muscles, leading to lack of urinary control and stress and urge incontinence.

- **Multiple sclerosis (MS)** is a progressive disorder in which the myelin sheath and underlying nerve fibers in the brain, eyes, and spinal cord are damaged or destroyed. About 80% of those with MS develop bladder control problems because the electrical impulses to and from the brain are interrupted.
- **Cerebrovascular accident (stroke)** results from vascular lesions of the brain causing neurological damage. About 40% of people with strokes suffer from urinary incontinence. Post-stroke incontinence may be more likely because of pre-stroke incontinence and other forms of urinary tract disorders.

Endocrine Conditions

Diabetes Mellitus

Diabetes mellitus is a disease of the pancreas that occurs when the pancreas cannot produce enough insulin to control glucose levels in the body (Type I) or where the body does not respond to the insulin that is produced (Type II), resulting in increased glucose levels in the blood and multiple associated health problems. A small percentage of people with Type I diabetes develop autonomic nervous system involvement that causes neurogenic bladder. About 6.5% of all women with urinary incontinence also have diabetes. As neurogenic bladder progresses there may be mild loss of the sensation of the bladder being full to complete bladder paralysis. In order to urinate, the person must strain to void and often dribbles urine. They may have urge, stress, or mixed incontinence, which worsens if the diabetes is not well controlled and the person suffers from thirst and the frequent need to urinate.

Review Video: Diet, Exercise, and Medications for Diabetes
Visit mometrix.com/academy and enter code: 774388

Cushing's Disease

Cushing's disease is a condition that results in over-production of corticosteroids from a neoplasm of the adrenal glands or of the anterior pituitary gland. In rare cases, some types of lung cancers may produce corticosteroids. Cushing's syndrome may result from medical use of corticosteroids. Cushing's disease/syndrome has many negative effects, including hypertension, obesity, weakness, glucose intolerance, and persistent polydipsia and polyuria. The constant thirst and need to urinate, coupled with weakness and other health problems, often lead to urinary incontinence.

Diabetes Insipidus

Diabetes insipidus is triggered by lack of antidiuretic hormone (ADH), which is stored in and released from the pituitary gland, or the inability of the kidneys to respond to ADH so that they are unable to conserve water as they filter the blood, resulting in excessive urination and extreme thirst. Patients drink copious amounts of water to compensate for fluid loss, often leading to the need to urinate every 1-2 hours and resulting urinary incontinence.

Obstruction

Obstruction within the bladder outlet is a frequent cause of overflow incontinence. The obstruction may be related to an enlarged prostate or a prolapse that compresses the urethra or interferes with the contraction of the detrusor muscle. Calculi, cancerous lesions, and strictures may also cause obstruction. Urethral trauma or sexually transmitted diseases may result in obstructive strictures of the urethra. When obstruction occurs, the part of the urinary tract proximal to the obstruction becomes distended and pressure builds, forcing the urine past the obstruction and often resulting in urinary stasis and infection. Chronic obstruction can cause permanent urinary tract damage. Upper urinary tract obstruction within the ureters or kidneys often causes pain and systemic reactions as hydronephrosis develops and the kidneys fail, but lower urinary tract obstruction of the bladder and/or urethra is more likely to present as urinary dysfunction with frequency, dribbling, hematuria, inadequate emptying, nocturia, and incontinence.

Pregnancy and Childbirth

Pregnancy and childbirth increase the risk of urinary and fecal incontinence, both during pregnancy from increased pressure exerted by the fetus and weakening of the pelvic floor muscles and after childbirth with a vaginal delivery, especially if forceps were used to aid in the delivery or if an episiotomy was done. Cesarean sections do not appear to result in post-partal incontinence. Older and multiparous women, especially after high-risk deliveries, are more likely to develop both urinary and fecal incontinence because of nerve damage sustained during childbirth as well as damage to the anal sphincter. The first vaginal delivery a woman has usually accounts for most of the damage to the anal sphincter, but subsequent births increase damage to the pudendal nerve, making fecal incontinence more common as the maternal age increases. Weakening of the vaginal walls and pelvic muscles can lead to prolapse, further causing urinary incontinence.

Effects of Incontinence on Males

Incontinence in males is much less prevalent than in females with only 3-11% of males affected, but this still means that 5 million men in the United States suffer from incontinence. Males have about half the rate of incontinence as women. Urge incontinence (40-80%) is the most common type, followed by mixed incontinence (10-30%), and only rare occurrences of stress incontinence (<10%), primarily because of the longer urethra in males. Stress incontinence, when it does occur, is usually the result of neurological injury or trauma, especially after surgery on the prostate. Urge incontinence is often related to bladder outlet obstruction causing bladder overactivity. It is also common with men who have Parkinson's disease, diabetes mellitus, stroke, or dementia. Overflow incontinence, often transient, is caused by blockage or weak contractions of the detrusor muscle. It is usually a result of prostatic hypertrophy or urethral stenosis related to scarring.

Normal Changes of Aging That Can Contribute to Incontinence

Normal changes of aging are physiological changes that take place, as people grow older. Most changes do not impact normal functioning although they may become more apparent under stress caused by physical exertion or illness. Some physiological changes can impact the urinary system:

- **Renal filtration** decreases, and the urine becomes less concentrated, so pH may be low even if dehydration is present. There is a loss of about 30-40% of functional nephrons in the kidney, decreasing the size of the kidneys and resulting in a decrease in the ability to concentrate urine. Excess potassium may be secreted, leading to dehydration.
- **Neurological changes due to degeneration** in the nerves or reflex arcs that control the bladder and sphincter muscles can cause frequency and urgency, leading to a decreased bladder capacity.
- **Muscle deterioration** can cause detrusor muscle of the bladder to lose contractibility, decreasing bladder capacity and preventing complete emptying of the bladder. Pelvic floor and sphincter muscles may atrophy, resulting in incontinence.
- **Prostatic hypertrophy** may cause obstruction of urinary flow and overflow incontinence.
- **Nocturnal urine production** increases, and this may result in nocturia and enuresis.

Stress Incontinence

Etiology

Stress incontinence is the leakage of urine during activities that apply pressure to a full bladder. When the stress on the bladder ends, the leakage ends. If the leakage continues after the pressure has been relieved, then the patient more likely has urge incontinence.

Stress incontinence is most often the result of urethral sphincter incompetence caused by weakened pelvic floor muscles and ligaments. This weakening causes the urethra, sphincters, and bladder neck to lose support and muscle tone and the urethra to rotate downward during episodes of stress, such as coughing or sneezing, overloading the urethral sphincters. When there is an increase in intra-abdominal pressure, it forces urine past the sphincters. The most common causes of this type of problem are related to trauma of childbirth causing damage to the sphincters or the pelvic floor muscles, loss of estrogen after menopause resulting in atrophy and loss of pliability of the urethra, and obesity, which causes chronic pressure to the pelvic floor muscles. Some muscle changes are common in the elderly, especially women. Stress incontinence in men is usually caused by neurological injury or trauma to the urethral sphincters, usually related to surgery on the prostate.

Having a **chronic cough** forces the patient to perform a bearing down type of activity, which applies pressure to the bladder and can cause some urine leakage.

Urethral hypermobility occurs when the urethra does not close properly, resulting in the leakage of urine. This is one of the main causes of stress incontinence. It is due to a weakening of the muscles in the pelvic floor, which occurs after vaginal deliveries. Urethral hypermobility may also occur after menopause when estrogen levels are low, causing the lining of the urethra to thin and not close properly. Treatment of stress incontinence involves performing exercises to help strengthen the muscles of the pelvic floor and the urethral sphincter.

Physical Causes

Physical causes of stress incontinence varies between females and males. In females, it results from one or more of the following:

- **Urethral hypermobility** is failure of urethral sphincter to close completely and the urethra being too mobile and out of normal position, related to weakening of the pelvic floor muscles. Urethral hypermobility is classified as Type I with incomplete closure of the bladder neck and urethra. With Type II, the bladder neck shifts position and a cystocele may develop.
- **Intrinsic sphincteric deficiency** is weakening of muscles around the bladder neck so the urethral sphincter cannot maintain adequate resistance for urinary continence. The bladder neck stays open when the bladder fills.
- **Denervation** related to trauma of childbirth, chronic cough, or lifting.

In males, stress incontinence is usually the result of trauma from surgical or radiation treatments for cancer of the prostate.

Functional Incontinence

Functional incontinence is characterized by leakage of urine because of the inability of the person to manage toileting or remove clothing for a variety of reasons. Management depends upon the cause.

- **Pain** may prevent people from attending to body functions, so adequate pain assessment and pain control must be initiated.
- **Dementia** may, in some cases, respond to medications. In other cases, the person may need the assistance of a caregiver to set up a program of scheduled, prompted voiding.
- **Inaccessibility** issues in the home may require modifications of bathrooms, including elevated toilet seats and safety bars. Bedside commodes or urinals may make toileting easier. Outside the home, accessible toileting facilities may need to be identified in advance.

- **Motor disability** must be dealt with according to disability. Sometimes assistive devices may be used. Clothes that are easy to remove, without buttons or zippers, may make toileting easier.

Environmental Causes

Environmental factors can have an impact on the ability of people, especially the elderly or disabled, to remain continent, resulting in functional incontinence:

- **Decreased mobility** may prevent people from being independent in toileting, and lack of assistance from caregivers can lead to inability to use toilet when needed.
- **Inaccessibility of toilet facilities**, such as no wheelchair accessible toilets or no assistive devices, including elevated toilet seats and safety bars, may be a barrier to toileting. Poor lighting may also be a factor for those who are visually impaired.
- **Restraints** can include clothes that are too tight or difficult to remove or physical restraints that preclude toileting. Restraining chairs or other types of restraints in nursing homes without adequately scheduled toileting can lead to incontinence.
- **Social attitudes** may prevent people from asking for the assistance that they need because some people feel ashamed or embarrassed, recognizing negative attitudes toward incontinence.

Urge Incontinence

Urge incontinence is usually the result of over-activity of the detrusor muscle of the bladder and hyperreflexia, resulting in inappropriate contractions of the detrusor muscle during the urinary storage stage. Usually, the bladder stretches to hold up to 550 mL of urine, with the urge to urinate occurring at about 200 mL, at which point, voluntary contraction of the bladder results in relaxation of the external sphincters and urination. With urge incontinence, contractions are unrelated to the amount of urine in the bladder. These premature contractions cause increased pressure in the bladder accompanied by an intense urge to urinate. When bladder pressure exceeds urethral pressure, urge incontinence occurs. This condition may be caused by lesions of the upper motor neurons, stroke, spinal cord tumors, neuromuscular disorders (Parkinson's disease, multiple sclerosis), and transverse myelitis. Urinary infections may also cause urge incontinence although infrequently. The cause for most urge incontinence is idiopathic.

Physical Causes

Urge incontinence occurs when bladder pressure exceeds urethral sphincter pressure. People feel the urge to urinate followed by immediate urination before they are able to reach a toilet. Causes relate to the detrusor muscle.

- **Detrusor hyperactivity with hyperreflexia** involves the detrusor muscle contracting involuntarily during the storage phase, causing a sensory perception of urgency, and forcing urine past the sphincters, leading to decreased bladder volume. The cause may relate to strokes, cervical stenosis, Parkinson's disease, urinary infection, or neoplasms.
- **Detrusor hyperactivity with impaired contractile function (DHIC)** results from involuntary contractions that may be ineffective to empty the bladder. This condition is characterized by overactive detrusor contractions during the storage phase but underactive contractions during urination, resulting in both frequency and residual urine in bladder. It is common with neurological impairment from trauma or disease, such as Parkinson's or multiple sclerosis.
- **Urinary infection** or other conditions that irritate the bladder may trigger contractions.

Reflex Incontinence

Reflex incontinence is a type of urge incontinence related to impairment of the neurological system. The transmission that is necessary in the spinal and brainstem reflex loops is impaired, so sensations of bladder fullness, sphincter control, and coordination of detrusor muscle and sphincter muscles are also impaired. Bladder emptying is impaired and usually incomplete. Reflex incontinence is common in patients with stroke, brain tumors, Parkinson's disease, multiple sclerosis, advanced dementia, and those with suprapontine or suprasacral spinal cord injuries. Physiologically, there are primarily two conditions that result from the neurological damage:

- **Detrusor hyperreflexia** involves aberrant contractions of the detrusor muscle without the sensation of needing to urinate. This can cause incontinence at unpredictable times and with no warning.
- **Dyssynergic contractions of the urethral sphincter muscle** are often present as well, resulting in urinary obstruction, which in turn causes a distended bladder with large residual urine volumes.

Overflow Incontinence

Overflow incontinence is the leakage of small amounts of urine both day and night from a distended bladder overflowing. The bladder fills normally, but cannot properly empty, leading to frequency and dribbling. Overflow incontinence is usually the result of bladder neuropathy with diabetes mellitus being a common cause of a neurogenic bladder. Tumors of the spine, meningomyelocele, and disk disorder may also result in bladder neuropathy. Overflow incontinence occurs when there is either a nonfunctioning detrusor or outlet obstruction from prostatic hypertrophy, urethral stricture, neoplasm, or urethral obstruction resulting post-operatively from a pubovaginal sling. A non-functioning detrusor may be the result of an underlying neurologic disease, such as Parkinson's disease, that essentially paralyzes the muscle. It may also result from an atonic bladder caused by chronic over-distention that has made the bladder lose muscle tone. Obstruction may be caused by a cystocele as well. Some medications also may interfere with bladder contractibility. With overflow incontinence, the bladder fills normally, but does not properly empty until the pressure becomes sufficient to force urine from the bladder or past an obstruction.

Physical Causes

Physical causes of overflow incontinence include:

- **Detrusor underactivity** results in a bladder that cannot adequately contract. Diabetes Mellitus is a common cause of nerve damage, resulting in a neurogenic bladder. Other causes are tumors of the spine, meningomyelocele, and disk disorders. Underactivity may also be the result of a neurological disorder, such as Parkinson's disease. Anticholinergics and opioids are also a cause.
- **Bladder outlet obstruction** may be caused by a cystocele, prostatic hypertrophy, urethral stricture, trauma from a sling procedure, or a fecal impaction.
- **Detrusor-sphincter dyssynergia** is a loss of coordination resulting in the sphincter contracting when the detrusor muscle contracts, creating an outlet obstruction. This condition often results from spinal cord lesions that interrupt neurological pathways and reflex arcs.

Post-Prostatectomy Incontinence

Post-prostatectomy incontinence is common with some studies showing that 30-47% reported some incontinence, ranging from dribbling to full emptying of the bladder. There are a number of reasons, and more than one may contribute to a person's incontinence:

- **Trauma to urethral sphincter** during the surgical procedure may result in transient or permanent stress incontinence with coughing, straining, or physical activity that increases intra-abdominal pressure.
- **Detrusor hypertrophy** occurs preoperatively as the bladder tries to compensate for urinary blockage with increasing muscle mass and pressure during contractions. After surgery, the bladder continues to contract with too much pressure for the urethra to prevent urination, resulting in urge incontinence. Hypertrophy may also cause frequency and sometimes enuresis. If this condition occurs with urethral trauma, it results in mixed incontinence,
- **Nerve damage** may affect the ability of the bladder to store low volumes of urine, resulting in dribbling.

Nocturnal Enuresis

Nocturnal enuresis is involuntary urination during sleep after the age of 5 while remaining continent during the daytime. In **primary enuresis**, the person may never have consistently stayed dry at night from childhood, sometimes lasting throughout adulthood. There appears to be a genetic factor involved in some cases. With primary enuresis, urinary output increases during the night. **Secondary enuresis** is adult onset, and there are a variety of causes:

- Chronic urinary retention with urethral obstruction causes overflow incontinence.
- Urinary tract infections may cause bladder spasms.
- Congestive heart failure may result in peripheral edema that resolves at night with an increase in urinary output.
- Neurological disorders, such as Parkinson's disease, may cause bladder spasms and chronic retention with overflow.
- Prostatic hypertrophy or cancer may cause obstruction
- Abnormalities of anatomy.
- Sleep apnea

People who suffer from urge or overflow incontinence during the daytime often also suffer from nocturnal enuresis.

Bowel Dysfunction

Colon Motility Disorders and Intractable Constipation

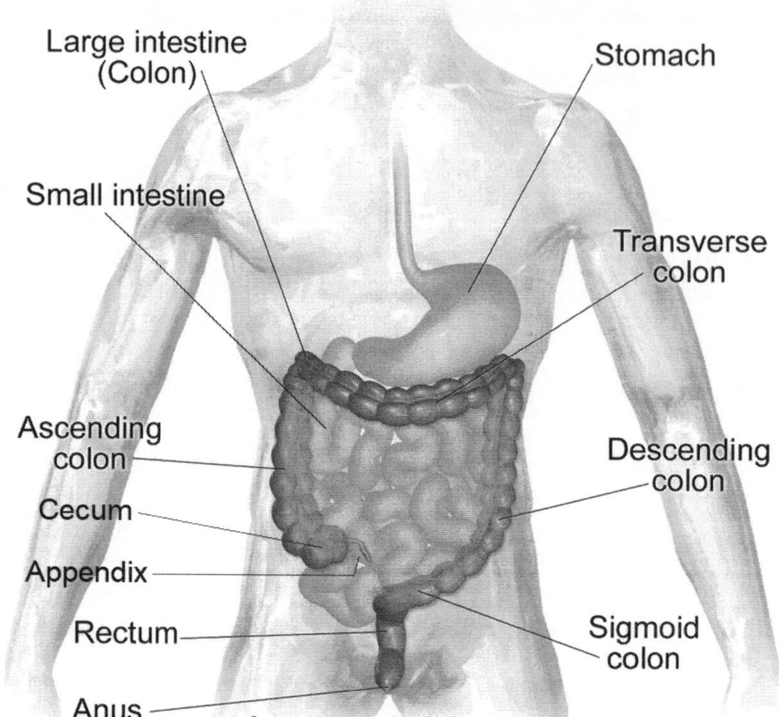

Anatomy of Colon

Colon motility disorders may involve the colon, pelvic floor muscles, and anal sphincter muscles. Many of these disorders so impair functioning that intractable constipation results. These disorders may include:

- **Abnormal contractions of the colon** may be spastic and ineffectual in pushing the stool through the bowel so that the stool becomes increasing dry and impacted.
- **Dysfunction of nerves or muscles of the colon** because of a neuromuscular disorder may cause an absence of contraction that delays movement of stool through the colon or allows only incomplete bowel movements. Severe constipation and impaction may result.
- **Functional obstruction of anal sphincters** results in the stool becoming trapped in the rectum because the anal sphincters partially or completely fail to relax to allow defecation.
- **Dyssynergia of pelvic floor muscles** prevents coordination of relaxation and contraction that propel stool from the rectum and through the anus, preventing normal fecal evacuation.

Contributing Factors to Bowel Dysfunction

Contributing factors to bowel dysfunction range from those things that can be corrected and others that require compensation:

- **Dietary factors** include insufficient fiber and fluids as well as foods that cause diarrhea, constipation, and gas.
- **Clinical conditions** such as hemorrhoids may cause pain that delays defecation. Surgical treatment of hemorrhoids, fistulas, or the rectum may create trauma and injury to the sphincters. Chronic diseases, such as irritable bowel syndrome and multiple sclerosis may be associated with bowel dysfunction. Dementia may result in the inability to manage toileting.
- **Delaying defecation**, often because of functional disability or dementia, is the leading cause of constipation, impaction, and fecal incontinence.
- **Pregnancy** can result in damage to anal sphincters, causing incontinence.
- **Medications** frequently cause constipation, but some, including antacids and antibiotics, may cause diarrhea. Laxative abuse causes laxative tolerance to develop.
- **Physical inactivity** decreases bowel motility and increases constipation.

Causes of Fecal Incontinence

Common causes of fecal incontinence include:

- **Constipation**: Chronic constipation causes stretching and weakening of intestinal and anal muscles. Weakened intestinal muscles slow down the passage of fecal material that forms impactions, and the weakened anal muscles prevent the rectal sphincter from closing. Chronic constipation may create a cycle of constipation/diarrhea, and stool leaks around impactions.
- **Chronic or severe diarrhea**: Inflammation and irritation from severe diarrhea with urgency can make it difficult to be continent of watery stools.
- **Injury to anal sphincter**: Usually related to damage during childbirth.
- **Neurological abnormalities/ injuries**: Congenital defects, such as myelomeningocele, can damage nerves and paralyze intestinal or anal muscles. Spinal cord injuries may also damage nerves.
- **Chronic laxative abuse**: Laxatives stimulate bowels to contract, causing irritation and cycles of constipation/diarrhea.
- **Surgical/radiation complications**: Rectal, prostate, or gynecological surgery may damage nerves or muscles controlling defecation. Radiation may cause scarring, inflammation, and stenosis.
- **Psychological/ psychiatric disturbances**: Severe mental or emotional problems may interfere with control of bodily functions.

Causes of Constipation and Impaction

Causes of constipation and impaction include:

- **Insufficient fiber** in the diet reduces bulk of stool, making it move more slowly through the colon.
- **Insufficient liquids** can make stools too dry and compact.
- **Lack of exercise** may decrease motility of bowel, slowing down the passage of stool and allowing more fluid to be absorbed.

- **Medications**, such as narcotic analgesics (codeine, meperidine, hydrocodone-containing drugs), antacids (Maalox, Mylanta), anticholinergics (tolterodine, oxybutynin, Donnatal), beta-blockers, (atenolol, propanolol), tricyclic antidepressants, iron supplements, calcium supplements, anticonvulsants (phenytoin), Antidiarrheals (diphenoxylate/atropine, bismuth subsalicylate) and diuretics (chlorothiazide, furosemide) can all result in constipation. Overuse of laxatives can result in a cycle of diarrhea and increasing constipation.
- **Irritable bowel syndrome** may be characterized by diarrhea, constipation, and impaction.
- **Pregnancy** with hormonal changes and pressure on the colon may lead to constipation.
- **Delayed toileting** for any reason, such as inaccessible toilets, travel, or pain about anus can cause people to delay defecation.

Risk Factors for Fecal Incontinence

Common risk factors for fecal incontinence include:

- **Age**: Fecal incontinence is most common among people who are elderly and may suffer from other health problems, including urinary incontinence.
- **Sex**: Women suffer more from fecal incontinence than men because women often suffer damage to the sphincter after childbirth, especially as scar tissue forms after episiotomies or muscles weaken after multiple childbirths.
- **Neurological damage**: Congenital or acquired neurological defects are frequently associated with fecal incontinence. Additionally, people with chronic disorders, such as diabetes mellitus or multiple sclerosis may lose the ability to control defecation because of progressive neuropathy.
- **Dementia/Alzheimer disease**: Late-stage Alzheimer disease is characterized by both fecal and urinary incontinence.
- **Physical disability**: Congenital or acquired physical disabilities may lead to fecal incontinence for many reasons. People confined to wheelchairs might find toilet access difficult. People may not be able to express the need to defecate. Others may not be able to physically manage toileting without assistance.

Rectoceles and Enteroceles

Rectoceles **(rectal prolapses)** occur when the muscles between the wall of the vagina and rectum weaken and the rectum prolapses or protrudes into the back wall of the vagina. **Enteroceles** occur similarly when the small bowel protrudes into the upper vaginal wall. Both can result from damage to the lower pelvic muscles from childbirth-related trauma, pelvic surgery, or muscle weakness attributed to aging. Rectoceles and enteroceles may occur together after hysterectomy. They can be felt as a bulging mass in the vagina. Enteroceles rarely after bowel habits, but rectoceles can cause chronic constipation and difficulty in passing stool because of weakening of the muscles, contributing to fecal incontinence. Untreated, rectoceles can cause inflammation, ulcerations, and fistula formation. Pessaries may reduce the prolapse. Surgical repair may not correct all symptoms, especially underlying damage to muscles, and can result in surgical trauma to the rectum or sphincters, adding to the risk of incontinence.

Intestinal Infections

Intestinal infections may be caused by numerous varieties of bacteria (*E. coli, Campylobacter, Clostridioides difficile, Shigella)*, viruses (*Rotavirus, Cytomegalovirus)*, fungal parasites (*Microsporidia)*, protozoan parasites (*Giardia intestinalis, Entamoeba histolytica), and* helminth parasites (*Strongyloides stercoralis, Angiostrongylus costaricensis*). While the pathogens may be different, most result in acute or chronic enteritis and/or colitis. Diarrhea is a common finding with almost all infections of the intestine, and in about 40% of cases, the etiologic agent cannot be identified. Infections can result in inflammation and ulceration of the mucosal lining as well as damage to the muscular layer. Recent studies have indicated that some individual with acute enteritis will develop chronic abdominal pain and altered bowel habits, a condition now referred to as **postinfectious irritable bowel syndrome (IBS)**. Some enteric infections will result in long-term effects on the neurological and muscular functions of the bowels, sometimes resulting in alterations of bowel habits, reduced sensation, and incontinence.

Fistulas

Fistulas are abnormal tunnel-like openings usually between two organs, or from an organ to the surface of the skin. Fistulas involving the anus, rectum, or vagina and the perineal tissue can result in damage to intestinal and pelvic floor muscles, nerves, and sphincters. Anorectal fistulas, the most common type, usually result from an abscess and may have one or more tunnels connecting the rectum and the skin around the anus. Fistulas may also result from trauma, disease, or radiation. Fecal incontinence is common with fistulas because of the extensive inflammation and tissue involvement. Fecal material may leak from the fistula as well as the anus. Surgical repair may require much dissection, especially if there are multiple tracts and the origin is high in the rectum, and can lead to cutting the muscles of the anus as well as the formation of scar tissue, further contributing to fecal incontinence.

Neuromuscular Conditions

Neuromuscular conditions may include a wide range of neurodegenerative disorders, traumatic nerve injuries, toxic metabolic disorders of the peripheral nerves and muscles, and autoimmune neuromuscular disorders, many of which result in damage to muscles and nerves, affecting bowel function, including the following:

- **Parkinson disease**, a chronic progressive neurodegenerative disease, affects movement. Both voluntary and involuntary muscle control may be compromised, sometimes resulting in loss of sphincter control and fecal incontinence.
- **Multiple sclerosis (MS)** is a progressive disorder in which the myelin sheath and underlying nerve fibers in the brain, eyes, and spinal cord are damaged or destroyed. The nerves that control bowel movements can be affected, causing constipation and fecal incontinence.
- **Muscular dystrophy (MD)** is a term designating a group of genetic disorders that cause progressive weakening and atrophy of muscles. Any level of the gastrointestinal tract may be involved, and fecal incontinence is a frequent problem with some types of MD.

Cancer

Several kinds of cancer are associated with fecal incontinence with the treatment rather than the cancer often being the precipitating factor. Colon and rectal cancer may remove or damage the muscles or nerves that control defecation. **Radiation therapy** may further cause weakening of the intestinal muscles or damage to the nerves. This damage may result in temporary fecal incontinence, but in some cases, the damage may be so severe that the fecal incontinence remains permanent. In some cases, cancer outside of the gastrointestinal tract may precipitate fecal incontinence. **Cancerous lesions** of the brain or spinal cord may both be related to bowel dysfunction and loss of bowel control because of cognitive defects or neurological damage. Because the nerves carry impulses from the brain to the spinal cord to the bowels, lesions involving these nerves or parts of the brain that controls these nerves can lead to incontinence.

Bowel Obstruction

Bowel obstruction is a mechanical blockage at any level of the small or large intestines. Bowel obstruction can be the result of a disease process, such as Crohn's disease, a cancerous lesion, herniation, foreign bodies, or a fecal impaction. Obstruction may be caused by something inside the lumen of the intestine, which is creating a blockage; within the wall of the intestine, which is narrowing the lumen; or outside of the intestine (such as a volvulus), which is causing a compression blockage. Complete or incomplete obstruction can result in ileus, cramping, distention, constipation and paradoxical or overflow diarrhea. Chronic constipation with impaction is a common cause of obstruction in the elderly or those who are bedridden and unable to manage their own toileting. Distention of the intestine brought on by the impaction can interfere with peristalsis, worsening the condition, and increasing the incidence of fecal incontinence.

Bowel Trauma

Bowel trauma comprises both blunt and penetrating abdominal wounds.

- **Blunt** trauma is usually the result of accidents or assaults and can result in intestinal injury through compression or deceleration. Compression of the lumen can stretch or perforate the bowel wall. Blunt injuries to the transverse colon, sigmoid colon, or cecum are common. Deceleration forces can tear the bowel and result in ischemia.
- **Penetrating** trauma is usually secondary to knife, shrapnel, or gunshot wounds and can involve minor to catastrophic injury. War injuries such as bomb and grenade trauma can involve both blunt and penetrating trauma. Small bowel wounds are easily misdiagnosed but can result in peritonitis and ileus. Bowel dysfunction, including fecal incontinence can result from both blunt and penetrating wounds, depending upon the degree, type, location of injury, and medical or surgical intervention. Bowel trauma may also be caused by laparoscopic injury during surgical procedures, especially gynecological endoscopy.

Encopresis

Encopresis is the voluntary or involuntary passage of stool in places or manners that are inappropriate for a child, 80% of whom are male, 4 years or older. There are two types: **retentive encopresis**, which accounts for about 80% of those affected, and **non-retentive**, which accounts for the other 20%.

- **Retentive encopresis** is characterized by a history of long term, painful constipation and the development of overflow diarrhea. The chronic constipation causes distention of the rectum and stretching of both the internal and external anal sphincters; as a result, the child may no longer feel the urge to defecate, so stool eventually leaks from the rectum, causing chronic fecal incontinence.
- **Non-retentive encopresis**, usually involving passage of normally formed stools on a daily basis, does not involve constipation or bowel abnormalities, except in a small subset that may have irritable bowel syndrome, but is generally a behavioral/psychological problem.

Endocrine Conditions

Endocrine conditions are those related to endocrine glands, which are glands that secrete hormones into the blood stream, through which the hormones reach the cells of the body.

- The **thyroid gland**, in the neck, regulates body metabolism. Hypothyroidism occurs when the gland does not produce enough hormones, causing multiple symptoms, including chronic constipation. Hyperthyroidism, on the other hand, causes increased bowel movements. Both conditions can lead to fecal incontinence, especially in the elderly and weak.
- The **adrenal glands**, located on top of the kidneys, produce adrenaline and cortisol. Addison's disease occurs with inadequate production of cortisol, affecting almost every body system. One symptom is chronic diarrhea, which coupled with weakness and vomiting, can lead to fecal incontinence.
- The **pancreas** produces insulin. Insufficient insulin leads to Type I diabetes mellitus, for which diabetic neuropathy is a complication causing autonomic and peripheral nerve changes, resulting in poor rectal tone, perianal hypoesthesia, and fecal incontinence.

Pelvic Pain Syndrome and Fecal Incontinence

Pelvic pain syndrome is characterized by persistent or recurrent episodes of pelvic pain that is associated with urinary, sexual, bowel, or gynecological dysfunction despite lack of evident infection or other pathology. The pain must be continuous or recurrent for 6 months or more. In males, it is often associated with perineal (including anal) and penile pain (often referred to as chronic prostatitis). The distribution and intensity of pain can vary considerably from one individual to another and may involve many different organs and structures. The particular aspects of pelvic pain syndrome that relate to fecal incontinence are the anorectal pain syndrome, which relates to bowel dysfunction and **anismus**, which is pain related to defecation. Because the pain is so severe, people afflicted with the disorder may retain stool because of the pain associated with defecation, leading to chronic constipation, which further aggravates the condition and is a factor in fecal incontinence.

Types of Pelvic Organ Prolapse

Pelvic organ prolapse occurs when pelvic floor muscles weaken with age or trauma and cannot support the pelvic organs. The uterus is the only organ that can fall into the vagina. Other organs can push against and cause a protrusion in the wall of the vagina.

- **Cystocele** is the bladder falling toward the vagina, causing an anterior vaginal wall protrusion.
- **Urethrocele** is the urethra pushing against the anterior vaginal wall, near the vaginal orifice, often occurring with a cystocele and called a cystourethrocele.
- **Enterocele** is part of the small intestine falling into the space between the rectum and posterior vaginal wall.
- **Rectocele** is the rectum protruding into the posterior vaginal wall while a rectal prolapse is the rectum falling through the anus.
- **Uterine prolapse** is the uterus falling into the vagina.
- **Vaginal vault prolapse** is the top of the vagina falling in on itself after hysterectomy.

Colonic Inertia and Constipation

Colonic inertia is a condition resulting from neuromuscular disorders of the colon causing a marked delay in the movement of fecal material through the colon. Stool often remains in the ascending or transverse colon rather than progressing to the rectosigmoid area. There may also be a lack of urgency even when the stool in the rectum. Three or more bowel movements weekly are average, but, because of delay in passage of stool, the person with colonic inertia may defecate only about every 7-10 days. Other abnormalities may occur, such as delayed emptying of the stomach and a condition calls pseudo-obstruction of the small intestine with no blockage but symptoms of blockage. The cause of colonic inertia is not always clear, but sometimes the nerves and muscles are diseased. It can also be caused by chronic use of stimulant laxatives. Colonic transit studies help to diagnose the condition. Complete colonic inertia may require ileostomy.

Pelvic Floor Dysfunction and Constipation

Pelvic floor dysfunction is also referred to as functional outlet obstruction or outlet delay, occurs when the pelvic floor muscles that surround the rectum cannot contract properly or loose muscle tone. Essentially the pelvic floor muscles act as a sling for the rectum. With pelvic floor dysfunction, there is a non-neurogenic lack of coordination of the muscles. The muscles may not relax properly to allow the anal sphincter to open, so stool remains in the rectal vault. Even if colonic motility is normal and there is no delay in transit, chronic constipation and impaction can result. Stool in the rectal area presses on the bladder and urethra and increases urinary problems, so constipation needs to be managed carefully. Pelvic floor dysfunction can occur in both males and females, and in men it is usually called prostatodynia. Ano-rectal motility studies may be done to help with diagnosis.

Complications of Incontinence

Moisture-associated skin damage, a common complication of incontinence, is inflammation of the skin from frequent and prolonged exposure to liquid, such as urine or feces, resulting in erosion of the tissue. Irritation most commonly occurs in the perineal region and up the gluteal fold and down the inner thighs. Treatment includes controlling incontinence, use of barrier creams, and avoidance of alkaline skin cleansers or detergents.

Intertriginous dermatitis occurs when moisture develops or accumulates in folds of skin, such as under abdominal rolls, in the axillae, or under breasts. The tissue may become erythematous, itching, painful, and denuded. The skin must be kept clean and dry and exposed to air. Powder may help prevent moisture.

Fungal skin infection occurs when the irritation and moisture results in alterations of normal skin flora and overgrowth of fungi, such as *Candida.* The skin becomes red, weepy, and itching. Treatment includes identifying and treating underlying cause and topical antifungal.

Screening

Routine Urinary Screening

Routine urinary screening measures several components of urine to determine if there is an abnormality:

- **Color** should be pale amber. Concentrated urine is often dark. Blood in the urine will discolor urine red or brownish. Some medications change color of the urine.
- **Clarity** assesses the cloudiness of the urine. Normal urine should be clear. Other material in the blood, such as pus, blood, sperm, and mucous, can increase opacity.
- **Odor** should be faint. A foul odor may indicate infection, and concentrated urine may have a strong odor. Some foods, such as asparagus or fish, change the odor.
- **Specific gravity** should range from 1.005 to 1.035. Higher levels can indicate concentrated urine. Low levels may indicate dilute urine, diuretic use, or kidney disease.
- **Protein** should not be found in the urine. Its presence is a sign of kidney disease, heart failure, leukemia, mercury or lead poisoning, or preeclampsia.
- **pH** should range from 4.5 to 8.0. An alkaline (high) pH can be caused by urinary tract infections, diarrhea, or kidney infection. An acidic (low) pH may reflect lung disease, severe diabetes, diarrhea with dehydration, excessive alcohol intake, or starvation.
- **Glucose** should not be found in the urine and may indicate uncontrolled diabetes mellitus but may also indicate liver damage, brain injury, and some kinds of kidney disease.
- **Nitrites** in the urine are indicative of a urinary tract infection.
- **Leukocyte esterase** indicates that there are white blood cells in the urine, probably from a urinary tract infection.
- **Ketones** should not be found in urine and can indicate uncontrolled diabetes, a low carbohydrate diet, anorexia or bulimia, excessive alcohol intake, or fasting for 18 hours or more.

Microscopic Analyses

Microscopic analysis of urine involves placing the urine specimen in a centrifuge to separate out the sediment, which is then examined under a microscope:

- **Erythrocytes** should not be in the urine and may indicate inflammation, injury, or slight bleeding from strenuous exercise.
- **Leukocytes** in the urine usually are indicative of infection, cancer, or kidney disorders.
- **Casts** are caused from kidney disease that causes tiny tube-like plugs of material (red or white cells, protein, and fatty substances) to be flushed from the kidneys to the urine. The type of cast may help with diagnosis.
- **Crystals** should appear in small numbers. Some types of crystals or large numbers of crystals may be a sign of kidney stones or a metabolic disorder.
- **Bacteria** in the urine indicate an infection.
- **Fungi** in the urine indicate a yeast infection
- **Parasites** may migrate to the urinary system in some types of infestation.

Diagnostic Tests

Endoanal Ultrasound and Rectal Ultrasound

Endoanal ultrasound uses high frequency sound waves and a computer to visualize to a depth of 5 cm the structure of the sphincter muscles and surrounding tissue. It is used to diagnose perianal fistulas and abscesses and to assess sphincter damage related to fecal incontinence and for staging and follow-up of malignant infiltrations of sphincters with anal neoplasms.

The **procedure** is as follows:

- With the patient lying on the left side, a narrow, wand-like endoscopic probe with a transducer and a lubricated rigid plastic cone covering the end is inserted into the anal canal and pictures are viewed on a computer screen. The cone has a uniform diameter to prevent anatomical distortion.
- Patients may feel vibration during procedure.

Rectal ultrasound is a similar procedure in which an ultrasound probe with an inflatable balloon is inserted through a scope to the rectum. The balloon is inflated and images are taken. This test is used to evaluate rectal masses.

Renal and Bladder Ultrasound

Renal ultrasound uses high frequency sound waves and a computer to visualize the location, size, and shape of the kidneys and other urinary structures, such as the ureters. It is used to diagnose tumors, cysts, calculi, and abscesses as well as for placement of drainage tubes.

The **procedure** is as follows:

- Patient is placed in prone position on table.
- Clear gel lubricant is placed on skin over kidney area.
- The transducer is pressed against the skin and moved about the kidney area for scans.

Bladder ultrasound is often done at the same time as the renal ultrasound and the procedure is similar.

The **procedure** is as follows:

- Patient is given fluids prior to the test to ensure full bladder.
- Patient is placed in the supine position on the table.
- Scans are taken of full bladder as for kidney scans.
- Patient empties bladder.
- Additional scans of bladder area are done.
- Gel wiped from skin.

Anal Sphincter Electromyography

Anal sphincter electromyography (EMG) assesses muscle contractions to determine if the sphincter muscles are contracting properly. A normal EMG reading with manometry findings of low anal pressure can indicate a torn sphincter muscle. If the pelvic floor muscles and sphincter muscles are contracting paradoxically rather than in concert, electrical activity increases during simulated defecation rather than decreases. Drugs such as muscle relaxants, cholinergic and anti-cholinergic preparations can affect the outcome of the test and may need to be stopped prior to having the EMG.

The **procedure** is as follows:

- With patient lying on the left side, a small lubricated sponge or plug electrode is inserted into the anal canal. Alternately, needle electrodes may be used.
- Patient must lie still during the procedure or results will be affected.
- Electrical activity of the anal sphincter muscles is recorded on a computer screen while the patient tightens the sphincter muscles, relaxes, and pushes.

Balloon Expulsion Test and Pudendal Nerve Terminal Motor Latency Test

Balloon expulsion test assess the length of time it takes to expel an inflated balloon. A dysfunction in the anorectal area may result in prolonged expulsion time.

The **procedure** is as follows:

- With patient lying on the left side, a balloon is inserted into the rectum and inflated with water.
- The patient sits on the toilet and tries to expel the balloon as though defecating.
- The time needed to expel the balloon is recorded.

Pudendal nerve terminal motor latency test assesses the pudendal nerve and the delay between an electrical impulse and the corresponding muscle contraction. It is used to evaluate incontinence, rectal prolapse, and constipation.

The **procedure** is as follows:

- With the patient lying on the left side, a gloved finger is inserted into the anus. The glove contains a stimulating electrode. With the finger serving as a guiding probe, several electrical impulses are delivered and nerve conduction assessed.
- Mild discomfort may be felt with stimulation.

Cystometrogram

Cystometrogram (CMG) assesses bladder capacity and pressure and is used to diagnose incontinence, dysuria, or neurological disorders affecting bladder function.

The **procedure** (may vary) is as follows:

- After emptying bladder, patient is placed in supine position.
- A very small thin catheter is inserted into the bladder. It has a tiny filament inside that is connected to a computerized device or a cystometer.
- Sterile saline at room temperature is instilled into the bladder followed by instillation of warm water to evaluate thermal sensation.
- The fluid is drained and then water or carbon dioxide gas is instilled into the bladder in a slow controlled manner while patient reports first need to urinate.
- The patient coughs or performs other activities while bladder is full, and pressure readings are obtained.
- The patient urinates with sensor in place to record pressures for voiding cystometrogram.
- Another catheter may be placed in rectum to record pressures.
- Catheter(s) removed.

Urodynamic Testing

Urodynamic testing assesses bladder and sphincter muscles and the ability of the bladder and urethra to store and release urine. It diagnoses problems with urination, such as frequency, incontinence, dysuria, recurrent infections, frequent urge to urinate, and difficulty initiating stream of urine or emptying bladder.

- **Uroflowmetry** measures the flow rate of urine, including the speed of urination and the volume.
- **Post-void residual measurement** shows how much urine is left in the bladder after urination is completed.
- **Cystometry** assesses bladder capacity and pressure, including how full the bladder is when the urge to urinate is felt.
- **Leak point pressure** measures the bladder pressure at the point where leakage of urine occurs.
- **Pressure flow study** measures bladder pressure that is needed to urinate and the flow rate at different pressures.
- **Electromyography** measures activity of muscles in and around the urethral sphincter.
- **Video** with fluoroscopy shows filling and emptying of bladder.

VLLP

Valsalva Leak point pressure (VLPP) measures the pressure at which bladder pressure overcomes urethral resistance without contraction of the detrusor muscle of the bladder wall. A decreased leak point pressure suggests stress urinary incontinence.

The **procedure** (may vary) is as follows:

- Position patient in supine position.
- A 6-10 Fr. Microtip pressure transducer catheter is inserted into the bladder. There may be a urinary sensor that slides over the catheter and up to the urethral meatus to measure any drops of urine.
- A rectal probe monitors intra-abdominal pressure.
- The patient sits or stands during the testing.
- The bladder is instilled with saline or contrast material at 50 mL/min to a total of 200 mL.
- Patient asked to make a progressive Valsalva motion, bearing down with a closed glottis, until incontinence. Patient may also be asked to cough.
- Procedure repeated for comparison measurements and catheters removed.

Urethral Pressure Profile

Urethral pressure profile is a graph recording the intraluminal pressure of the entire length of the urethra. The profile assesses the function of the urethra during filling cystometry.

- **Urethral pressure**: The pressure of fluid needed to open a urethra.
- **Maximum urethral closure pressure**: The maximum pressure exerted by the urethra as indicated on the profile.
- **Functional profile length**: The length of the urethra (in females) where the pressure is greater in the urethra than the pressure inside the bladder.
- **Pressure transmission ratio**: The relationship (in percentage) between an increase in urethral pressure as a response to stress and the simultaneous increase in bladder pressure.

- **Abnormal leak point pressure**: The pressure at which bladder pressure overcomes urethral resistance without contraction of the detrusor muscle.
- **Detrusor leak point pressure**: The lowest pressure of the detrusor muscle at which urinary incontinence occurs without contraction of detrusor muscle or increased abdominal pressure.

Cystography

Cystography is a urinary diagnostic test that uses x-rays or fluoroscopy to examine the bladder. The test may be used to determine how well the bladder empties and whether there is a vesicoureteral reflux (backflow of urine to the kidneys). It can assess the cause of hematuria, chronic urinary tract infections, obstructions, and urinary incontinence.

The **procedure** is as follows:

- Patient may be given laxatives or enema before cystography.
- Patient will empty bladder before procedure.
- Patient is placed in supine position on x-ray table.
- Catheter is inserted into bladder and contrast dye is injected through the catheter, which is then clamped.
- X-rays or fluoroscopy are done.
- Patient may have to change positions for different views.
- Catheter removed.
- For **voiding cystography**, x-ray or fluoroscopy will be done while the patient urinates. The patient may be allowed to sit up if unable to urinate in supine position.

Uroflowmetry and Pad Test

Uroflowmetry is a non-invasive test that plots the flow rate of urination over time and is used to assess function of the bladder and sphincters. During normal urination, the first stream starts slowly, speeds up and then slows down again as the bladder nears empty. This pattern may alter with urinary tract obstruction.

The **procedure** is as follows:

- Patient urinates into special funnel attached to a measuring instrument.
- The instrument calculates rate of flow in seconds, amount of urine, and time of urination.
- The uroflowmeter converts the information into a graph.

Pad test is a non-invasive method of assessing frequency and severity of urinary incontinence.

The **procedure** is as follows:

- Patient is asked to keep a bladder diary.
- Pre-weighed absorbent pads are provided to patient.
- The pad is worn until leakage occurs, and then removed, sealed in a Ziploc-type bag, labeled with date and time.
- Pads are weighed and urine output estimated according to weight.

Intravenous Pyelogram

Intravenous pyelogram is an x-ray of the kidneys and ureters after injection of a contrast dye used to diagnose kidney disease or disorders of the urinary tract. This test may be completed with a CT scan of the kidneys. IVP helps to evaluate kidney function and diagnose bladder or ureteral stones, injury, trauma, and tumors.

The **procedure** is as follows:

- The patient may be given a laxative and enema or suppository before test.
- An intravenous line will be inserted.
- The patient is positioned in supine position on x-ray table.
- A KUB x-ray is taken.
- Contrast dye is injected into the IV.
- To help with visualization, a band may be placed around the waist.
- X-rays are taken at timed-intervals over about 30 minutes as dye progresses through the urinary tract.
- Patient may be asked to change positions.
- Patient empties bladder.
- A final x-ray is taken.
- Intravenous line is removed.

Antegrade Pyelogram

Antegrade pyelogram is an x-ray used for the diagnosis of obstruction in the kidneys and ureters. Fluoroscopy or ultrasound may be used to locate kidney and ureters.

The **procedure** is as follows:

- Patient may be given prophylactic antibiotics before or after procedure.
- An intravenous line may be inserted for emergencies.
- Patient lies prone on the x-ray table.
- Area of lower back will be cleansed and sterile drapes applied.
- A local anesthetic is injected at dye injection site.
- Under ultrasound or fluoroscopy, a needle is inserted into the renal pelvis. A wire may be fed through the needle to allow for placement of catheters or tubes.
- Contrast dye is injected into the renal pelvis.
- A number of x-rays are taken at timed intervals as the dye progresses from the kidney through the ureters.
- Needle removed or tubes placed.
- Urine is monitored for volume and hematuria.

Retrograde Pyelogram

Retrograde pyelogram is an x-ray with contrast dye that provides visualization of the organs of the urinary tract. It is usually performed during a cystoscopy. The retrograde pyelogram is done to diagnose a suspected obstruction of the upper urinary tract or for placement of ureteral stents or catheters.

The **procedure** is as follows:

- Patient may be asked to fast for a number of hours.
- Laxatives or cleansing enemas may be done as preparation.
- The patient may receive a sedative.
- An intravenous line may be inserted for emergencies.
- Patient will be positioned in supine position on the x-ray table with feet in stirrups.

- An endoscope is inserted through the urethra and into the bladder to examine the bladder.
- Catheters may be inserted into ureters and contrast dye injected through catheters. Endoscope is removed.
- X-rays are taken at timed intervals.
- Catheter is removed.

KIDNEY SCAN

Kidney scan is done after administration of a radioactive substance (radionuclide), usually technetium or iodine, which is absorbed by normal kidney tissue. The radioactive substance emits gamma radiation that is detected by a special scanner that converts the information into computerized pictures. Areas with uptake of the radioactive material are called "hot spots," and areas with fewer uptakes are "cold spots," indicating abnormal tissue. The scan is used to diagnose tumorous lesions, hematomas, abscesses, cysts, or enlargement of the kidney and to assess renal function and circulation.

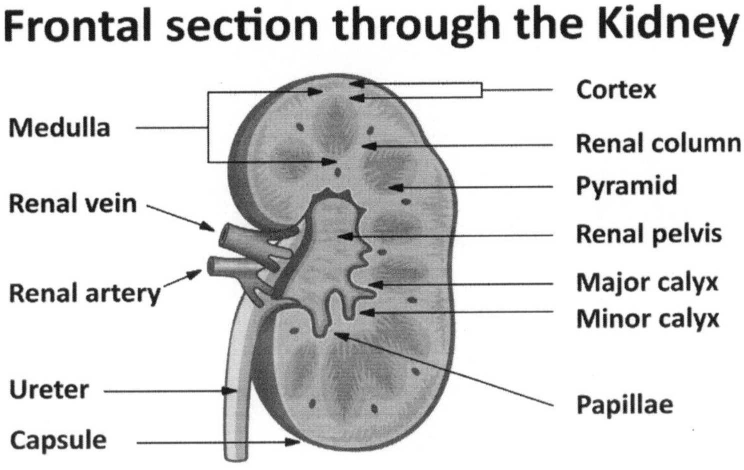

The **procedure** is as follows:

- Patient may be asked to drink fluids prior to scan.
- An intravenous line is started.
- The radioactive material (radionuclide) is injected into the IV.
- Patient may be asked to lie or sit without moving during the scan.
- Patient may receive other medications, such as a diuretic or ACE inhibitor during procedure.
- IV is removed on completion of scan.

KIDNEY, URETER, AND BLADDER (KUB) X-RAYS AND POST-VOID RESIDUAL URINE MEASUREMENT

Kidney, ureter, bladder (KUB) x-rays assess the urinary system as well as other structures of the abdominal area. They may be done to diagnose tumorous lesions, obstructions, and obstruction.

The **procedure** is as follows:

- No special preparation is needed.
- Depending upon the type of equipment, the x-rays may be taken standing or lying down, and from various positions.

Post-void residual urine measurement measures the amount of urine remaining in the bladder after the patient urinates and attempts to empty the bladder. It is used for diagnosis of neurogenic bladder, incontinence, bladder retention, and other urinary problems.

The **procedure** is as follows:

- The patient is placed in supine position and women usually with feet in stirrups.
- A small straight catheter is inserted into bladder to drain residual urine.
- Alternately, a bladder ultrasound with a B-mode (grayscale) sector scan may be done to estimate urine volume. Studies have shown that trans-vaginal ultrasounds are less accurate.

Cystoscopy

Cystoscopy assesses the urethra, bladder, and associated structures using an endoscope. It is used to diagnose urinary problems, such as cancer, retention, infections, obstruction, strictures, and bleeding. Tissue biopsy as well as irrigations or instillations may be done through the endoscope.

The **procedure** is as follows:

- Patient may be asked to fast or have a special diet before test.
- Patient may need to stop anticoagulants or aspirin therapy before test.
- The procedure may be done under a local anesthesia or with conscious sedation.
- An intravenous line is inserted.
- Patient is positioned in supine position with feet in stirrups.
- A topical anesthetic gel is placed in urethral meatus with a catheter.
- The cystoscope is inserted through the urethra into the bladder.
- Sterile water or saline may be instilled in the bladder to allow better visualization.
- A biopsy or urine specimen may be obtained.
- Cystoscope is removed.

Prostate/Rectal Sonogram

Prostate/rectal sonogram uses ultrasound technology with sound waves and computers to assess the size, shape, and location of the prostate, rectum, and surrounding structures. A transducer with a Doppler probe may be used to assess circulation of the prostate. This sonogram is used to diagnose prostatic cancer, especially after blood tests that show an elevated prostate-specific antigen (PSA). It may also be used to diagnose or stage rectal cancer.

The **procedure** is as follows:

- Patient may be given a small cleansing enema to clear rectum of fecal material prior to sonogram.
- Patient lies on examining table on the left side with knees drawn toward chest.
- A digital rectal exam may be performed.
- The transducer wand is lubricated and inserted into rectum and then rotated for visualization of the rectum and the prostate.
- A whooshing sound may be heard while Doppler is used. Wand is removed and gel wiped from skin.

Q-Tip Test and Provoked Stress Test

Q-tip test measures mobility and axis position of the urethra to assess urinary incontinence in women.

The **procedure** is as follows:

- Patient lies in supine position.
- Cotton swab (Q-tip), sterile and lubricated with anesthetic gel, is inserted through the urethra to the bladder and then pulled back to the bladder neck.
- Supine, patient strains as though urinating, and straining and resting angles of the swab are measured.
- Standing, the patient again strains and angles are measured.
- A positive result is a Q-tip angle of 30 degrees or more at maximal straining, indicating urethral hypermobility.

Provocative stress test is a cough test of urinary incontinence for women.

The **procedure** is as follows:

- Patient with full bladder in supine position with legs apart coughs, and leakage of urine confirms stress incontinence.
- Patient then stands with one leg on stool and holds pad or paper towel over perineum and coughs. A wet stain confirms stress incontinence.

Electromyogram of the Bladder

Electromyogram (EMG) measures activity of muscles in and around the urethral sphincters and measures coordination between the bladder and the urethra. EMG is used for spinal cord injuries and neurogenic bladder.

The procedure is as follows:

- The patient is in supine position.
- A catheter may be inserted into the bladder.
- Electrodes are placed. There are 3 types: Skin electrodes require skin clean and shaved; electrodes are taped in place around the urethra for females or on the lower abdomen, and between the scrotum and anus for males. Needle electrodes are inserted directly around and into the sphincter muscles for females and through the skin in the perineal area for males. Anal plug electrodes are inserted into the rectum.
- Patient is asked to contract and relax muscles, and electrical activity is recorded on a graph.
- Normal saline or water may be instilled into bladder and patient asked to urinate.
- Catheter and electrodes are removed.

Colonic and Nuclear Transit Studies

Colonic transit studies are x-rays showing how long food takes to go through the intestines. For 1-2 days, the patient ingests gelatin capsules containing small plastic radiopaque markers that can be visualized on x-ray. The gelatin dissolves and the plastic passes, with digested food, through the intestine. After 5-7 days, an abdominal x-ray is taken and the plastic markers are counted in different parts of the intestine. The counts show if there is a delay. In normal evacuation, all markers are expelled. If there is colon inertia, the markers may remain scattered about the colon, suggesting neuromuscular problems. With pelvic floor dysfunction, the markers may accumulate in the rectum.

Nuclear transit studies are similar but a small amount of radioactive material is dissolved in milk or fruit juice and ingested. Images are taken after 6 hours and daily for 4 days, 10 minutes from a large camera scan overhead and 10 minutes from below.

Anal Manometry

Anal manometry is an assessment of anal sphincter function, often used to evaluate the reason for chronic constipation or fecal incontinence. The test measures the pressure of the sphincter muscles, the degree of sensation in the rectum, and whether the neural reflexes that control normal bowel movements are intact.

The procedure (about 30 minutes) is as follows:

- The lower bowel is cleansed, usually with Fleet enemas about 2 hours before the assessment and food is restricted during this time.
- With patient lying on left side, a balloon catheter is inserted into the rectum. A machine connects to the catheter to measure pressure.
- The balloon is inflated in the rectum to simulate a feeling of fullness and the need to defecate to test neurological response of the reflex pathways.
- Pressure measurements are taken while the patient tightens, relaxes, and pushes with the anal sphincter muscles, simulating holding stool and expelling stool.

Ano-Rectal Manometry

Ano-rectal manometry is motility studies to evaluate the function of the nerves and muscles of the anus and rectum. In order to perform measurements of pressure, a small flexible tube with sensors is inserted through the anus into the rectum. A balloon may be inflated in the rectum to test pressures. The person is asked to do such things as tightening or relaxing the anal sphincter muscles while the sensors measure the changes in pressure generated by the muscles. These studies can assess whether the muscles of the anus and muscles are working normally or are impaired. With impairment, the muscles cannot coordinate to effect defecation, causing obstruction with resulting constipation. This condition is similar to pelvic floor dysfunction. Tests may show an inadequate sphincter response to rectal distention. Ano-rectal motility defects are common after radiotherapy for pelvic malignancies. Manometry may also be done to assess Hirschsprung's disease and idiopathic megacolon.

Defecography and Colonic Motility Studies

Defecography is a type of barium enema, with some modifications. It assesses the process of defecation and shows abnormalities in the anatomy of the rectum and pelvic floor muscles. A thick barium paste is inserted rectally, and then x-rays are taken as the person defecates. The barium outlines the physical structures and shows changes that occur in the pelvic floor muscles during evacuation.

Colonic motility studies measure the contraction pressures of the muscles of the colon. The procedure is done with colonoscopy. Sensors in the long 1/8-inch diameter manometry tube that is passed through the colon measure the pressure. Abnormal activity of the nerves and muscles will result in a pattern of abnormal colonic pressures. This test is useful for diagnosing colonic inertia and determining both cause and treatment for chronic constipation. Excessive contractions may be treated with medications, but complete colonic inertia may require colectomy and ileostomy.

Medical Procedures to Evaluate Causes of Constipation

Medical procedures to evaluate causes of constipation should be preceded by a careful history as this may help to define the type of diarrhea and guide the choice of diagnostic procedures. Most tests are necessary only for severe constipation that does not respond to treatment. Medical diagnostic procedures may include the following:

- **Physical exam** should include rectal exam and abdominal palpation to assess for obvious hard stool or impaction.
- **Blood tests** can identify hypothyroidism and excess parathyroid hormone.
- **Abdominal x-ray** may show large amounts of stool in the colon.
- **Barium enema** can indicate tumors or strictures causing obstruction.
- **Colonic transit studies** can show defects of the neuromuscular system.
- **Defecography** shows defecation process and abnormalities of anatomy.
- **Ano-rectal manometry studies** show malfunction of anorectal muscles.
- **Colonic motility studies** measure the pattern of colonic pressure.
- **Colonoscope** allows direct visualization of the lumen of the rectum and colon.

Physical Assessment and Tools

External Urogenital Exam

The external urogenital exam for males requires examination of the scrotum, testes, spermatic cords, and penis.

Inspect for any obvious abnormality, such as difference in size of testes, curvature of penis, discolorations, lesions, or mites. The scrotum is often slightly asymmetric with the left testicle lower than right. Note circumcision or intact prepuce. Check for inguinal hernias.

Palpate the scrotal skin for sebaceous cysts or other lesions. Gently palpate each testis between thumb and first 2 fingers for enlargement, masses, or tenderness. Testes should feel smooth and rubbery. The epididymis at the top of each testis should be smooth and nontender. Palpate each spermatic cord beside the penis and above each testis and note swelling or nodules. Slight tenderness is normal. Palpate the penis shaft for lesions or tenderness. Check the external urethral meatus for signs of inflammation or discharge and milk for discharge if necessary. Probe the inguinal ring around base of penis.

Physical Examination of the Skin

The skin, the largest organ in the body, is composed of 3 layers (epidermis, dermis, and subcutaneous tissue) and contains nerves, vessels, glands, and hair follicles. Some changes are normal signs of aging and don't represent pathology: diminished hair, liver spots, seborrheic keratoses, wrinkles, and spider angiomas.

Inspect by observing skin color for rashes, erythema, discoloration (hypopigmentation or hyperpigmentation), or cyanosis. Observe for plaques, ecchymosis, urticaria, nodules, nevi, macular spots, or chances. Note the size, shape, color, and character of any lesions as well as any discharge, odor, or necrosis.

Palpate the skin to feel the temperature for signs of inflammation (warm) or decreased circulation (cool). If rash is present, gently stretch the skin and palpate rim of lesions. Gently run fingers across skin to assess texture, dryness, or moistness. Pinch skin gently to observe for skin turgor and elasticity. Apply both light and heavier pressure to skin to check for sensory deficits.

Rectal Exam

The rectal exam is approached differently for males and females. Males usually stand for the exam and may lean slightly against the examining table. Females usually have the exam while on the examining table with feet in stirrups or lying on their side. The exam in done with a lubricated gloved finger inserted into the rectum while the other hand may press against the abdomen. Having the person bear down during the exam relaxes the external sphincter.

Inspect the perianal area, noting any internal or external hemorrhoids, fissures, skin tags, perianal fistulas.

Palpate upward, to both sides, and posteriorly to feel for masses or prolapse of the rectum. For examination of males, palpate anteriorly to examine for enlargement or nodules of the prostate. For females, a combined rectovaginal exam may be done to examine the uterus, cervix, and ovaries.

Usually, the stool on the glove is examined and may be tested for occult blood.

PELVIC EXAM

The pelvic exam is done with the woman on the exam table and feet in stirrups.

Inspect vulva with a bright light, and check pubic hair for nits or lice. Separate labia to inspect for swelling or lesions, such as venereal warts. Examine skin folds for ulcerative lesions, and retract clitoral hood to look for periclitoral lesions. Note if hymen is intact. Check position of the urethra and note any redness, swelling, or discharge. Check the Skene's glands next to the urethra.

Palpate the labia majora for masses. Bartholin cysts are felt in the middle or lower part of the labia majora.

Digital exam is done with 1 or 2 fingers in the vagina, palm upward, and the other hand compressing downward externally. Press the urethra upward against the pubic bone and note any tenderness that could indicate urethritis. Then insert finger(s) deeper and press bladder against pubic bone. Note pain that can indicate cystitis.

ANAL WINK AND BULBOCAVERNOSUS REFLEX

Anal wink **(anocutaneous reflex)** is the reflexive contraction of the anus in response to gentle stroking or stimulation of the skin around the rectum. It occurs in both females and males. Pulling the penis elicits the response in males as well; at one time, this response was believed indicative of sexual abuse, but that has been disproved. Failure of this response indicates that there in an interruption in the reflex arc in the sensory or motor nerves.

Bulbocavernosus reflex is the reflexive contraction of the anus in response to natural or electrical stimulation of the bulbocavernosus muscle of the penis. Both the bulbocavernosus and the ischiocavernosus contract during the rigid stage of erection, resulting in a suprasystolic pressure within the penis and causing the anal sphincter to contract, presumably to prevent leak of flatus or fecal material during coitus. Failure of the reflex is indicative of an interruption or defect in the reflex arc.

EVALUATING ODOR AND OTHER ABNORMAL STOOL CHARACTERISTICS

Odor and other abnormal stool characteristics should be noted as part of an evaluation of diarrhea or other bowel dysfunction:

- **Foul-smelling light grey, oily or frothy stool** may relate to malabsorption problems, such as decrease in bile, resulting in undigested fat (steatorrhea).
- **Heavy stools with high fat content** may to relate malabsorption, intestinal, or pancreatic disorders.
- **Floating stools** are related to malabsorption or excessive flatus as stools float because of increased air or gas in the stool.
- **Excessively foul-smelling stool** may be related to food intake or bacteria in the bowel.
- **Ammonia smelling stool** may be related to bacteria in stool or insufficiently digested nitrogen in foods.
- **Sulfur smelling stool** may be related to foods high in sulfur (cabbage, broccoli)
- **Mucus in stool** indicates irritation of the intestinal lining, such as from irritable bowel syndrome and ulcerative colitis. Bacterial infections, such as *Campylobacter* and *Shigella* may also produce mucus.

Stool Color

Stool color is directly affected by disease, foods, fluids, and amount of bile in the stool. Stools may normally vary in color, including all shades of brown and green-tinged:

- **Green stool** may be caused by leafy vegetables or green dye in foods. If stools are diarrhea, the bile may not have broken down as the stool moved quickly through the colon, causing green color.
- **Clay-colored stool** may indicate lack of sufficient bile or use of antidiarrheals, such as Kaopectate.
- **Black tarry stool** is often a sign of digested blood from upper gastrointestinal tract or from iron supplements, black dye (licorice), or Pepto-Bismol.
- **Red or bloody stool** may be a sign of bleeding in colon or rectum or caused by red dye in foods, beets, or tomato products.
- **Orange stool** may be caused by medications (rifampin) or beta-carotene in pills or foods, such as apricots, carrots, sweet potatoes, pumpkin, and mangoes.
- **Bright yellow stool** may indicate bile obstruction.

Incontinence Symptom Profile

An incontinence symptom profile helps to confirm the severity and pattern of incontinence. It also includes management strategies. The following factors are assessed:

- **Amount of leakage** may range from small amounts to full emptying of bladder.
- **Frequency** may range from normal (about 6 x daily) to every 1 or 2 hours.
- **Nocturia** may be present or absent.
- **Enuresis** may be present or absent.
- **Stream** may be normal, weak, difficult to start, or intermittent.
- **Sensation** of incontinence may be missing or related to strong urge.
- **Bladder emptying** may be complete or incomplete. Post urination dribbling may occur.
- **Mobility impairment** may interfere with toileting.
- **Medications** may impair awareness or bladder control.
- **Depression/dementia** can affect ability to control body functions.
- **Pain** may interfere with toileting or prevent people from emptying bladder.
- **Management** may include incontinence pads, disposable underwear, pessaries, dietary modifications, environmental modifications, and scheduled urination.

Stress Incontinence, Urge Incontinence, and Mixed Incontinence

Stress incontinence is characterized by small involuntary amounts of urinary leakage, usually without sensation. It occurs during the daytime, especially during physical activity that increases intra-abdominal pressure, such as coughing, laughing, bending, heavy lifting, exercising, or sneezing. Bladder capacity is normal and bladder usually empties completely on urination. There is generally no nocturia.

Urge incontinence is characterized by moderate to large amounts of involuntary urinary leakage caused by the sudden urge to urinate and the inability to hold the urine until able to reach a toilet. It is associated with frequency and nocturia more than two times nightly as well as small bladder capacity. Enuresis may occur.

Mixed incontinence is usually a combination of stress and urge incontinence with both small involuntary amounts of urinary leakage during activities as well as moderate to large amounts with the urge to urinate. Bladder capacity may be small and there is usually nocturia and possibly enuresis.

Overflow Incontinence and Functional Incontinence

Overflow incontinence is characterized by usually small leakages of urine, similar to stress incontinence, but resulting from pressure on an overdistended ladder. There is often difficulty initiating flow, requiring straining with a weak urinary stream so that urination can take longer than normal. There may also be dribbling after urination because bladder has not emptied. The person may feel the frequent need to urinate because the bladder feels full.

Functional incontinence is characterized by leakage of urine because of inability of the person to manage toileting or remove clothing for a variety of reasons. Some people may be constrained by pain. Some people with dementia, or those taking medications that cause sensory impairment, are not aware of the need to urinate. Sometimes, barriers, such as no wheelchair accessible toilets, may be the cause. Generally, bladder and urinary functions are normal for the person's age and condition.

Diarrhea

Diarrhea is passing liquid or semi-formed stool more frequently than is normal for an individual, often accompanied by abdominal cramping, distention, and sense of urgency to defecate. Severe diarrhea may occur hourly. Diarrhea should be characterized according to color, odor, consistency, and frequency. Diarrhea may be acute or chronic.

- **Acute diarrhea** generally has a sudden onset and may be related to medications such as chemotherapy, irritating foods, gastrointestinal organisms, and stress. Diarrhea may be very watery or bloody and may be accompanied by flatus. Acute diarrhea usually responds to Antidiarrheals or is self-limiting within a few days.
- **Chronic diarrhea** lasts longer than 3 days and is usually the result of a long-term disease process, such as Crohn's disease, or trauma, such as from radiation therapy. It may also result from dietary irritation or from overuse of constipation, in which case there may be a cycle of constipation followed by diarrhea.

Constipation and Impaction

Constipation is a condition with bowel movements less frequent than normal for a person, or hard, small stool that is evacuated fewer than 3 times weekly. Food moves through the gastrointestinal from the small intestine to the colon in semi-liquid form. Constipation results from the colon, where fluid is absorbed. If too much fluid is absorbed, the stool can become too dry. People may have Abdominal distension and cramps and need to strain for defecation.

Fecal impaction occurs when the hard stool moves into the rectum and becomes a large, dense, immovable mass that cannot be evacuated even with straining, usually as a result of chronic constipation. In addition to abdominal cramps and distention, the person may feel intense rectal pressure and pain accompanied by a sense of urgency to defecate. Nausea and vomiting may also occur. Hemorrhoids will often become engorged. Fecal incontinence, with liquid stool leaking about the impaction is common.

IAD

Incontinence-associated dermatitis (IAD), also known as perineal dermatitis, is the breakdown of skin expressed as inflammation, redness, or erosion, and causes a painful, itching, or burning sensation. This breakdown is due to the skin's continual contact with urine or stool. In some cases,

IAD can lead to a secondary bacterial skin infection. Fungal infections can also occur from incontinence associated dermatitis. To prevent this, it is important that the patient or their caregiver keep the skin clean and dry. The use of thick barrier creams should be avoided. If the condition worsens, it can lead to total skin breakdown and the development of pressure ulcers as the skin becomes macerated from exposure to urine. If necessary, absorbent briefs or pads should be used to wick moisture away from the skin and prevent the development of incontinence associated dermatitis. Seams and rough edges from these products should also be kept from the skin to prevent chafing or further irritation from rubbing. Patients should be educated to contact their physician if they should develop any signs of skin breakdown.

Assessment Tools Relevant to Continence and Associated Risk Factors

Urinary Incontinence Severity Index and Timed Up and Go

Assessment tools available to support the continence care nurse include:

- **Urinary Incontinence Severity Index**: This simple two-question screening tool is used to screen for urinary incontinence, track symptoms, triage patients, and document severity:

Q1 How often do you experience urinary leakage?	Q2 How much urine do you lose each time?
0 = Never	1 = drops or very little
1 = less than once per month	2 = small splashes
2 = one to several times per month	3 = more
3 = one to several times per week	
4 = every day	
Scoring: 1-2 slight; 3-6 moderate; 8-0 severe; 12 very severe.	

- **Timed up and go (TUG)**: This procedure is used to evaluate functional mobility, screen for risk of falls, assess balance and gait, and monitor progress. The patient stands from a chair with armrests, walks 3 meters, and turns, walks back, and sits back down. Those requiring >13.5 seconds indicates some risk for falls: Scoring: 7-10 seconds is normal for young, healthy adults, 10-19 seconds is typical of independent mobile older adults, 20-29 seconds indicates some functional limitations, and ≥30 indicates high risk of falls.

Fecal Incontinence Severity Index

The Fecal Incontinence Severity Index is a matrix that provides information about the type of incontinence and the frequency, helping with evaluation and treatment. Types include:

- **Flatus** incontinence is characterized by uncontrolled flatulence often exacerbated by activity that increases bowel motility.
- **Mucus** incontinence occurs in inflammatory bowel disease in response to irritation of the mucous lining of the bowel. Mucus may also be produced in response to fecal impaction. Mucus may be thick or watery.
- **Liquid stool** in the form of diarrhea can be difficult to contain, especially chronic diarrhea or leakage around impaction. Liquid stool may be watery, bloody, or purulent, depending upon the cause.
- **Formed stool** may be expelled, especially with neurological damage or damage the anal sphincter.

Patients are asked to indicate the frequency of these incidents by selecting one of the following:

- 2 or more times a day
- Once daily
- 2 or more times weekly
- Once weekly
- 1-3 times monthly
- Never

Bristol Stool Form

The Bristol Stool Form is named for Bristol University in England, where it was designed as a general description of stool constancy or form. The form is often given to people when they do a bowel diary so that they can more clearly identify for healthcare providers what types of stools they are passing.

The scale has descriptions and pictures to help people identify the correct type of stool:

- **Type 1** is separate small hard lumps of stool that are difficult to pass.
- **Type 2** is sausage-shaped lumpy stool.
- **Type 3** is sausage-shaped and lumpy but with cracks on the surface.
- **Type 4** is long, smooth, soft, snake-like stool.
- **Type 5** is soft blobs of stool that are easily passed and have clear-cut edges.
- **Type 6** is mushy, fluffy pieces of stool with uneven ragged edges.
- **Type 7** is watery stool that is entirely liquid with no solid pieces.

Continence Care: Intervention and Treatment

Stress, Functional, and Urge Incontinence Management

MANAGEMENT STRATEGIES FOR STRESS INCONTINENCE

There are a number of management strategies for dealing with stress incontinence, and the starting procedure depends on the level of incontinence and the motivation the person has to deal with the problem. Exercise alone may be enough for some people to control incontinence; others may need surgery:

- **Kegel exercises** can be used to strengthen the pelvic floor muscles and the "knack" to prevent incontinence.
- **Absorbent pads** may be used to contain leakage.
- **Urethral plugs** can be inserted into the urethra to block the urethra or **urethral patches** can be applied to seal the urethra externally.
- **Pessary** may relieve symptoms by elevating the angle of the urethral sphincter.
- **Weight loss** to relieve pressure on pelvic floor muscles may help.
- **Medications**, such as estrogens and adrenergic agents may increase control.
- **Surgical procedures** include the sling procedures, needle suspensions, and retropubic colposuspension, and injectable bulking implants.

THE KNACK

The knack is the use of precisely-timed muscle contractions to prevent stress incontinence. It is the practice of squeezing up before bearing down. The knack is a preventive use of Kegel exercises. Women are taught to contract the pelvic floor muscles right before and during events that usually cause stress incontinence. For example, if a woman feels a cough or sneeze coming, she immediately contracts the pelvic floor muscles and holds until the stress event is over. This contraction augments support of the proximal urethra, reducing the amount of displacement that usually takes place with compromised muscle support, thereby preventing incontinence. It is particularly useful if used before and during stress events, such as coughing, sneezing, lifting, standing, swinging a golf club, or laughing. Studies have shown that women who are taught this technique for mild to moderate urinary incontinence and use it consistently are able to decrease incontinence by 73-98%.

VAGINAL WEIGHTS/CONES FOR REHABILITATION OF PELVIC FLOOR MUSCLES

Vaginal weights are tampon-sizes cones that are inserted into the vagina during Kegel exercises to provide weight training and resistance for the pelvic floor muscles for stress incontinence. The stainless-steel cones come in sets of 5 in several weights (20-70 grams). They are usually coated with plastic and have a retrieval cord, like a tampon. Another type cone unscrews so that different weights can be placed inside. A test to determine correct size is to start with the weight that can be held for one minute. In the beginning, usually the lightest weight cone is inserted into the vagina, requiring the pelvic muscles to tighten to hold it in place. When the person can hold the lightest cone in comfortably, she moves up to the next size. Exercise with the vaginal weights is usually done two times a day for 15 minutes until the heaviest weight can be held.

PESSARIES

Pessaries are plastic or silicone removable prosthetic devices that are placed in the vagina for management of pelvic muscle support defects, such as cystocele and rectocele. They are also frequently used for stress incontinence. There are a wide variety of pessaries, and they are fitted to the individual. A pelvic exam is done prior to fitting a person for a pessary. Fitting sets are available to help the healthcare provider pick the right size, as the correct fit is crucial if the pessary is to be comfortable and provide needed support. Some pessaries are intended for self-care, and can be removed daily, weekly, monthly, (depending upon the type) washed with soap and water, and reinserted. Others are removed, cleansed, and reinserted periodically by a healthcare provider. In general, pessaries should not be left in place for more than 4 months at a time to ensure that there are no complications.

TYPES

Types of pessaries range from simple rings to inflatable balls. Different types are used for different disorders.

- **Ring/ring with support** is for 1st and 2nd degree uterine prolapse and cystocele.
- **Donut** is for 3rd and 4th degree uterine prolapse and vaginal vault prolapse.
- **Gehrung (arched U-shaped)** is for 2nd, 3rd, and 4th degree cystocele and rectocele.
- **Gellhorn (rigid and flexible)** is for 3rd and 4th grade uterine prolapse and must be removed prior to sexual intercourse.
- **Cube** is for 3rd degree uterine prolapse and must be removed daily.
- **Hodge** (with/without knob) is for mild cystocele.
- **Inflato-ball** supports prolapsing vaginal structures, is inflatable, and must be removed daily.
- **Shaatz** is for mild cystocele and uterine prolapse.
- **Incontinence dish and ring (with/without support)** is placed at base of bladder to support bladder neck and compress urethra to prevent stress incontinence.

PROCEDURE FOR FITTING

Fitting a pessary may require trial and error to arrive at the correct size and style. The type of pessary is determined by the problem the pessary is intended to correct and the type of muscle weakness or prolapse present.

- Pelvic exam performed.
- Average size pessary, usually in a simple style, inserted and checked for fit and effectiveness.
- A smaller or larger pessary may be inserted until the correct fit obtained, with the largest comfortable pessary the optimum choice for effectiveness.
- A finger must pass easily between the vaginal wall and the pessary.
- If treatment is for stress incontinence, the person coughs to test for urinary leakage.
- Person stands, sit, performs Valsalva maneuvers, and squats to make sure that the pessary remains in place.
- Person urinates to ensure there is no pressure that prevents urination.
- Person instructed regarding care and return visit to check placement.

CONTRAINDICATIONS AND COMPLICATIONS

Contraindications for a pessary include infection, such as vaginitis. Because most pessaries are made of silicone or latex, some people may have allergic response, especially to latex. Patients should not be fitted with a pessary if they are noncompliant and may not do follow up care.

Complications may occur, especially if the pessary is not cared for properly:

- **Vaginal discharge and odor** may be treated with acidic vaginal gel (Trimo-San) or vinegar douche.
- **Vaginal ulceration** may occur in post-menopausal women with atrophic vaginal mucosa. Estrogen cream can be used with pessary.
- **Embedding of pessary** may occur with a neglected pessary. Estrogen cream may help to decrease inflammation and allow removal, but surgical removal may be necessary. Fistulas may develop in severe cases.
- **Herniation of cervix and lower uterus with incarceration** can happen if a ring pessary is not fitted properly, causing herniation through the open center. Surgical repair may be needed.

Medical Devices for Women for Incontinence

Medical devices that are available for women to use to control incontinence stop the flow of urine by blocking the urethra. They are quite effective for many women.

- **Urethral plugs** are available in different types, but all are inserted into the urethral meatus. One type is inflatable with a balloon that prevents leakage. FemSoft is a typical one-use disposable plug. It looks like a tiny tampon but is a fluid-filled insert that seals the urethra. It is removed to urinate, and then a new plug is inserted. Plugs are fitted to the individual and may cause infection.
- **Urethral patches** are small multiple-use foam pads with gel adhesive. They are placed over the urethra to create a watertight seal and absorb small leakages if necessary.
- **Tampons** are intended for menstrual flow, but some women find that tampons provide pressure against the urethra, preventing mild incontinence.

Prompted Voiding to Promote Continence

Prompted voiding is a communication protocol for people with mild to moderate cognitive impairment. It uses positive reinforcement for recognizing being wet or dry, staying dry, urinating, and drinking liquids.

- Ask people every 2 hours (8 am to 8 pm) whether they are wet or dry.
- Verify if they are correct and give feedback, "You are right, Mrs. Brown, you are dry."
- Prompt people, whether wet or dry, to use the toilet or urinal. **If yes**, assist them, record results, and give positive reinforcement by praising and visiting for a short time. **If no**, repeat the request again once or twice. If they are wet, and decline toileting, change and tell them you will return in two hours and ask them to try to wait to urinate until then.
- Offer liquids and record amount.
- Record results of each attempt to urinate or wet check.

Urge Incontinence

Management strategies for urge incontinence are primarily conservative because surgical treatment has a high rate of morbidity:

- **Bladder training**, a behavioral therapy, has an improvement rate of about 75%. Scheduled urination should be done, gradually increasing time between urinations, along with strategies to delay urination. People who have dementia or caregivers may need prompted urination in order to maintain a schedule.
- **Fluid management** involves maintaining adequate fluid intake but decreasing fluids in the evening.
- **Reducing caffeine** and other bladder irritants may reduce contractions.
- **Medications** that cause bladder contractions should be reviewed as these may need to be discontinued or changed in order to control the incontinence.
- **Medications** include anticholinergics, such as tolterodine and oxybutynin and bladder relaxants, such tri-cyclic antidepressants, such as imipramine and dicyclomine. Medications are usually given only if behavioral therapy is unsuccessful. Medications with about a 46% rate of improvement have proven less effective than behavioral modifications

Reflex Incontinence

Management strategies for reflex incontinence are similar to those for urge incontinence, often with medication and catheterization:

- **Behavioral therapy** with scheduled urination to prevent distention and frequency, double voiding to prevent residual urine, use of the Credé maneuver to stimulate contraction of the bladder, and "trigger" voiding.
- **Absorbent pads or briefs** may be necessary to contain leakage.
- **External catheters** may be used by males instead of absorbent protective materials.
- **Intermittent clean catheterization** or long-term catheterization may be needed in order to empty the bladder if other methods fail.
- **Medications** such as tolterodine and Ditropan are used to control the overactive bladder and decrease contractions.
- **Neuromodulation/sacral nerve stimulation** with implantable neural prosthesis suppresses detrusor hyperreflexia through electrical stimulation of the sacral nerves.
- **Botulinum toxin** injections may be used to paralyze the bladder and sphincter muscles, but they must be repeated as the results are not long lasting.

Bladder Training

Bladder training usually requires the person to keep a toileting diary for at least 3 days so patterns can be assessed. There are a number of different approaches:

- **Scheduled toileting** is toileting or a regular schedule, usually every 2 to 4 hours during the daytime.
- **Habit training** involves an attempt to match the scheduled toileting to a person's individual voiding habits, based on the toileting diary. This is useful for people who have a natural and fairly consistent voiding pattern. Toileting is done every 2-4 hours.
- **Prompted voiding** is often used in nursing homes and attempts to teach people to assess their own incontinence status and prompts them to ask for toileting.

- **Bladder retraining** is a behavioral modification program that teaches people to inhibit the urge to urinate and to urinate according to an established schedule, restoring normal bladder function as much as possible. Bladder training can improve incontinence in 80% of cases.

Bladder Retraining to Promote Continence

Bladder retraining usually takes about 3 months to rehabilitate a bladder muscle weakened from frequent urination, causing a decreased urinary capacity. A short urination interval is gradually lengthened to every 2-4 hours during the daytime as the person suppresses bladder urges and stays dry.

- The person keeps urination diary for a week.
- An individual program is established with scheduled voiding times and goals. For example, if a person is urinating every hour, the goal might be every 80 minutes with increased output.
- The person is taught techniques to withhold urination: sitting on a hard seat or on a tightly rolled towel to put pressure on pelvic floor muscles, doing 5 squeezes of pelvic floor muscles, deep breathing, counting backward from 50.
- When the person consistently meets the goal, a new goal is established.
- The person maintains the use of a urination diary.

Biofeedback for Rehabilitation of Pelvic Floor Muscles

Biofeedback uses electronic or mechanical instruments to measure, process, and give feedback to people about neuromuscular activity. The perineometer, a pressure-sensitive vaginal probe, is the biofeedback device that helps women identify, train, and rehabilitate the pelvic floor muscles. A smaller device can be inserted into the rectum of men or women. The probes sense muscular activity. Occasionally, surface electrodes are placed around the rectum rather than using a probe. The therapy provides immediate visual or auditory feedback about the status of the muscle contractions. The biofeedback machine for pelvic floor muscles uses computer graphs or lights to indicate when the correct muscle is flexed. Some systems have both pressure and electromyograph channels, which allow various muscles to be monitored at the same time. Treatments are usually 20-30 minutes long and the average number of treatments is 6. Once a person has the ability to flex the correct muscles, Kegel exercises can be done.

Urge Suppression Techniques for Urinary Incontinence

Urge suppression techniques help suppress the urge to urinate, decrease frequency, and improve bladder tone and capacity:

- **Deep breathing** requires people to sit or lie down and take slow deep breaths in through the nose. Then exhalation is done through the mouth. The person is encouraged to concentrate, as in meditation, only on the breathing and to repeat the cycle 10 times.
- **Distraction** involves thinking of something else, such as counting backward or reciting out loud. Some people might keep a music player close at hand and listen to music.
- **Applying pressure** by sitting on a firm surface or on a rolled towel may apply pressure to the pelvic floor muscles and control urge.
- **Quick flicks** are the use of Kegel exercises. The person remains still, usually sitting or lying, and quickly tightens and relaxes the pelvic floor muscles about 10 times, in "flicks."

Other Incontinence Management Strategies

Overflow Incontinence

Management strategies for overflow incontinence include:

- **Behavioral therapy** with scheduled urination to prevent distention and frequency, double voiding to prevent residual urine, and use of the Credé maneuver to stimulate contraction of the bladder.
- **Absorbent pads or briefs** may be necessary to contain leakage.
- **External catheters** may be used by males instead of absorbent protective materials.
- **Intermittent clean catheterization** or long-term catheterization may be needed in order to empty the bladder if other methods fail.
- **Medications** for detrusor underactivity include cholinergic agonists, such as bethanechol. Males may get relief from outlet obstruction with alpha adrenergic blockers, such as doxazosin, prazosin, tamsulosin, and terazosin.
- **Treatment of prostatic hypertrophy** with surgery or medication, such as finasteride, which reduces the size of the prostate and relieves obstruction.
- **Bowel training**, including dietary interventions, to prevent chronic constipation and impaction will reduce associated overflow leakage.

Post-Prostatectomy Incontinence

Management of post-prostatectomy incontinence depends upon the reason for the incontinence.

- **Medications**, such as tolterodine and oxybutynin, relax bladder pressure with detrusor hypertrophy but are contraindicated in those with narrow angle glaucoma or with residual volume after urination. The Oxytrol patch (oxybutynin) may be used, usually with fewer side effects.
- External catheter, penile clamp, absorbent pads manage leakage.
- **Pelvic floor muscle exercises** may be helpful for mild stress incontinence.
- **Bladder pacemaker**, such as Interstim, requires a 2-stage surgical procedure where an electrode is placed by the main nerve controlling the bladder.
- **Artificial urinary sphincter** may be surgically implanted, with an inflatable cuff to control incontinence.
- **Male sling procedure** is done through a scrotal incision. Screws are placed in the pubic bone, to which the sling graft material (donor or synthetic) is attached with sutures that tighten the urethra. Studies show the failure rate is 20%, but 80% stay dry or improve.

Mixed Incontinence

Mixed incontinence includes both stress incontinence with impaired external sphincter control and urge incontinence with detrusor pressure exceeding sphincter pressure. Treatment deals with both problems and is primarily aimed at the most prominent type of incontinence:

- **Kegel exercises** strengthen the pelvic floor muscles and the "knack" may prevent stress incontinence.
- **Bladder training** with scheduled urination should be done, gradually increasing time between urinations, along with strategies to delay urination.
- **Fluid management** involves maintaining adequate fluid intake but decreasing fluids in the evening.
- **Reducing caffeine** and other bladder irritants may reduce bladder contractions.
- **Medications** that may cause bladder contractions should be reviewed as these may need to be discontinued or changed.
- **Absorbent pads** may be used to contain leakage.
- **Pessary** may relieve symptoms by elevating the angle of the urethral sphincter.
- **Weight loss** to relieve pressure on pelvic floor muscles may help.

Nocturnal Enuresis

Nocturnal enuresis may be managed in a number of different ways, depending upon whether the enuresis is primary or secondary, the severity, and whether there is also incontinence during the daytime.

- **Behavior modifications** such as bladder training, scheduled urination, fluid restriction, and dietary modifications as well as conditioning therapy with enuresis alarms may be helpful, especially for primary nocturnal enuresis.
- **Medications** such as antidepressants (imipramine) relax the bladder and tighten the urethral sphincter, desmopressin at bedtime reduces urinary production for 5-6 hours, and anticholinergics reduce instability of the detrusor muscle.
- **Neuromodulation** by sacral nerve stimulation may help voiding dysfunction.
- **Botulinum toxin** is a neuromuscular blocking agent that reduces detrusor overactivity.
- **Surgical treatment** includes clam cystoplasty, bladder augmentation to increase bladder capacity, and detrusor myectomy, which is removal of part of the outer muscle of the bladder to reduce the overactive contractions.

Nocturia

Nocturia is waking up one or more times during the night with the need to urinate. Some authorities believe that one event at night is within normal limits. Some people have to urinate 5 or 6 times at night. About 70% of cases of nocturia are related to over-production of urine at night. Nocturia is one of the most common causes of sleep deprivation. It affects about two-thirds of those aged 50-59. Studies have shown that nocturia more than 2 times nightly is strongly linked with depression. Treatment aims at reducing urination during the night:

- **Desmopressin** acts as an antidiuretic hormone that reduces volume of urine by increasing concentration and allows for about 5 hours of undisturbed sleep. It increases the first period of sleep by about 2 hours. Desmopressin is the primary treatment for nocturia.
- **Fluid management** by reducing fluids in the evening can help some people.

Overactive Bladder (Urgency/Frequency) Without Incontinence

Overactive bladder is a condition with urgency, frequency, and nocturia but without incontinence. The urge to urinate may be as frequent as every 20-30 minutes in extreme cases and, if nocturia is present, people may become sleep-deprived. If overactive bladder includes incontinence, it is known as urge incontinence, and the treatment is similar for both:

- **Anticholinergics (antimuscarinics)**, such as tolterodine and oxybutynin relax the bladder muscle and relieve the symptoms.
- **Pelvic floor muscle exercises**, such as Kegel exercises, vaginal weight training, as well as biofeedback or pelvic floor electrical stimulation done with the Kegel exercise program.
- **Behavioral modification** with bladder training that includes scheduled voiding with increasing time between urination and strategies to delay urination. Prompted urination may be needed for some people, especially those with dementia.
- **Fluid management** involves maintaining adequate fluid intake but decreasing fluids in the evening.
- **Reducing caffeine** and other bladder irritants may reduce contractions.

Obsessive Toileting

Obsessive toileting, as frequently as every 20-30 minutes, may occur with neurogenic bladder when people develop the fear that they will be incontinent. The goal is to stop the behavior and institute successful retraining.

- **Educate** person about bladder capacity, the normal capacity and the amount of urine in the bladder after repeated urinations (usually about 50-75 mL).
- An **ultrasound** scan may be used to check volume of urine in the bladder when person wants to urinate to show actual need.
- If bladder volume is under 100-150 mL, encourage person to **extend toileting time**. If the person has some dementia, it is important to stay with the person, giving assurance and support, until the urge to urinate eases.
- Try to **distract** the person by talking, playing music, engaging in activities.
- **Monitor fluids** as people may be drinking less in the mistaken belief it will reduce incontinence.

Detrusor Hyperactivity with Impaired Contractile Function

Detrusor hyperactivity with impaired contractile function (DHIC) results from involuntary contractions that may be ineffective to empty the bladder. This condition is characterized by overactive detrusor contractions during the storage phase but underactive contractions during urination, resulting in both frequency and residual urine in bladder. It is common with neurological impairment from trauma or disease, such as Parkinson's or multiple sclerosis. Some medications commonly used for hyperactivity (tolterodine and oxybutynin) can make DHIC, so treatment can be challenging. Conservative treatment is the most common:

- **Behavioral modification** with bladder training that includes scheduled urination, prompted urination if necessary, Credé maneuver, and double voiding may help with emptying bladder and reducing frequency. Diet modifications to eliminate bladder irritants and to control fluid intake may help control incontinence.
- **Clean intermittent catheterization** to completely empty bladder on a regular schedule can decrease or eliminate incontinence and is often necessary to prevent bladder distention.

Detrusor Sphincter Dyssynergia

Detrusor sphincter dyssynergia is a loss of coordination resulting in the sphincter contracting when the detrusor muscle contracts, creating an outlet obstruction. This condition results from spinal cord lesions interrupting neurological pathways and reflex arcs. Some treatments result in constant leakage and are not done for females because of the risk of skin irritation:

- **External catheters or penile clamps** may be used by males.
- **Intermittent clean catheterization** or long-term catheterization is often needed, especially for females, in order to empty the bladder.
- **Insertion of urethral stent**, such as UroLume, which is a mesh tube that holds the urethra open (for males), resulting in incontinence requiring external catheter.
- **Pudendal nerve block with 5% phenol** may be effective.
- **Intraurethral botulinum injections** help but must be repeated.
- **External sphincterotomy** enlarges the urethral sphincter in males, resulting in incontinence requiring external catheter.
- **Muscle relaxants** may be used to relax urethra.

Device Management and Absorptive Products

Environmental Modifications to Help Prevent Urinary Incontinence

Environmental modifications are those changes that make it easier for people to toilet and to prevent incontinence.

- **Bedside commodes** are useful at night if the bathroom is not near the bed. They can also be used during the daytime to make toilet access easier especially if there is no toilet on the same floor. They should be adjusted for height and easy to empty.
- **Urinals** are available for both men and women although male urinals are easier to use and generally more successful. They can be kept within arm's length.
- **Bedpans** can be used, if there are care providers. They are very difficult to use without assistance because they spill easily.
- **Doorknobs** may be replaced with levers to facilitate opening doors.
- **Elevated toilet seats** and **safety bars** in the bathroom may help people to get on and off of the toilet more easily.

Catheterization for Urinary Incontinence

Catheterization for control of urinary incontinence can be done in 3 different manners.

- **Clean intermittent catheterization** is used for spinal cord injuries and urinary retention. Catheterization is done several times per day, usually on a regular schedule about every 4 hours, using clean catheters. Sterile catheters may be advised for impaired immunity. Catheters must be cleansed properly and replaced as needed.
- **Indwelling Foley catheters** provide a closed, sterile system that is useful for urinary incontinence related to obstruction or urinary retention. Foley catheters may be inserted if people are too ill to care for themselves or to protect the skin. The catheters are usually changed monthly or as needed.
- **Suprapubic catheters** are inserted through a surgical opening in the lower abdomen. They are used for those who need long-term catheterization as they are more comfortable and have fewer problems than Foleys. The catheters are changed at least every month.

External Catheters and Penile Clamps for Men for Urinary Incontinence

External catheter systems are condom catheters that are available for men. They are usually made of latex or silicone and are attached to the penis shaft by adhesive, inflatable cuffs, or straps. They come in different sizes, and proper sizing is important to prevent constriction. They are disposable and usually only used for 24-49 hours. A drainage tube and leg bag or overnight bag is attached to the external catheter. Many men prefer these to disposable adult diapers.

Penile clamp is a device that is clamped on the penis to prevent incontinence. It is clamped about halfway down the penis shaft and has soft foam on the inside of the clamp. The clamp is released every 1-2 hours to prevent circulatory restriction and to allow for urination. It is very important that the clamp not be placed too tightly as it can cause strictures or skin breakdown, even necrosis.

Indwelling Catheters

Indwelling catheters are left in place for continuous urinary drainage either through the urethra or a suprapubic opening into the bladder. Foley catheters have double lumens, a larger for urinary drainage and a smaller leading to an inflatable balloon near the end of the catheter. There are various types:

- **Antibiotic coated catheters** are expensive catheters impregnated with antibiotics to discourage infection.
- **Coudé catheters** have a 45-degree angled tip, especially useful with enlarged prostate.
- **Silicone catheters** are thin walled, resulting in a larger lumen for drainage. They discourage protein and mucus buildup, preventing obstruction.
- **Silicone/Teflon coated latex catheters** have a coating to protect urethra from contact with latex.
- **Silver-coated catheters** have a bacteriostatic effect that decreases inflammatory response to catheter.

The smallest catheter that allows drainage is preferred; usually 12-18 Fr. Larger sizes can cause urethral irritation. Balloon size is usually 5 mL; 10-30 mL sizes are available but can interfere with urinary drainage and increase inflammation.

Problems Related to Catheters

Catheters are invasive devices that can result in a number of problems:

- **Spasms** are a normal reaction to the catheter and may cause some urinary leakage. Some burning may be felt as well.
- **Catheter loss** may occur because of strong spasms that expel it or it can be pulled out accidentally or intentionally. People with confusion often pull at the catheter.
- **Urinary leakage** may happen for a variety of reasons: spasms, infection, bladder irritation, over-inflated balloon, or catheter size too large.
- **Obstruction** may be caused by encrustations from mucus, crystallizations, or purulent material. The tip may become plugged with calculous material, especially if the urine is alkaline. Increasing fluid intake and acidifying the urine with 500-1000 mg per day may help.
- **Infection** is common because bacteria usually develop in 2-4 weeks after insertion. Bacteria may migrate up the catheter so hygiene is very important.

Containment Products for Incontinence

Absorbent Pads

Containment products vary in quality and type. Depends and Poise are brands that are widely available. The product needed relates to the degree of incontinence.

Absorbent pads are rated for size and degree of absorbency, light to heavy. Some women use panty liners, but these are less absorbent than urinary products and need to be changed frequently. Absorbent pads have fill, such as wood pulp or polymer, which binds with urine and changes it to a gel. The surface area wicks the urine to the absorbent layer so that the skin can stay dry, decreasing skin irritation. Absorbent pads usually have a plastic layer to prevent leaks and an adhesive strip on the back so that they can be placed inside panties or shorts and secured into position. There are pouch-type absorbent pads that fit over the male penis. Absorbent pads are most useful for stress incontinence or those with light to moderate incontinence.

Reusable Undergarments and Disposable Briefs

Containment products for moderate heavy urinary or fecal leakage vary, but all are intended to protect clothing and furniture as well as to give the user a feeling of confidence that incontinence will be contained.

- **Reusable undergarments/brief** are made with a fiber core of rayon or polyester and can be washed and reused. They may have a plastic covering on the outside. They are less expensive but also less convenient than disposables.
- **Disposable adult undergarments** include open-sided products with a belt around that can be worn alone or under panties or shorts. There are a number of different types of briefs. Most are paper products with elastic around the hips to accommodate different sizes, an absorbent center, and elastic gathering at the legs. Some are simple pull-ups. Overnight briefs may have an outside plastic lining for more absorbency. Some briefs are refastenable, which is useful for people who are bedridden.

Surgical Interventions

Surgical Procedures for Urinary Incontinence

Common surgical interventions in the treatment of urinary incontinence include the following:

- **Anterior bladder repair** releases the anterior vaginal wall from the bladder, folds the supportive tissue, and secures it to tighten the vaginal wall and repair prolapses.
- **Artificial sphincter** is a balloon reservoir, pump, and cuff encircling the urethra to manually inflate and deflate.
- **Injectable bulking implants** include collagen or silicone injected into tissue about the urethra, increasing bulk of the surrounding tissue and compressing the urethra.
- **Needle suspension** places stitches on side of bladder and attaches them to muscle tissue or pubic bone for support.
- **Percutaneous sling procedure** uses a piece of ligament, muscle tendon, or synthetic material to create a sling about the urethra to lift it to normal position.
- **Retropubic colposuspension** lifts the bladder neck and urethra by attaching bladder and urethra or the vaginal wall to other pelvic structures.
- **Tension-free vaginal tape procedure** uses a mesh-like synthetic tape under urethra to form a sling to lift it to normal position.

Artificial Sphincter

Artificial sphincter is a balloon reservoir and pump with a cuff encircling the urethra to manually inflate and deflate. The 3 components are filled with normal saline. This procedure is done when the urethral sphincters are non-functioning, and is used for both men, especially after radical prostatectomy, and women. For males, the pump is installed in the scrotum, the reservoir in the lower abdomen, and the cuff around the urethra near the bladder neck. For women, pump and reservoir are installed in the labia. The pump activates by squeezing or pressing on a button. When the cuff is deflated, the saline drains into the reservoir and then returns to the cuff after button is re-pressed. The procedure is done under a general or spinal anesthesia. A Foley catheter is inserted during surgery and is left in for a few days. The artificial sphincter is not inflated for about 6 weeks, giving the tissue time to heal.

Anterior Bladder Repair

Anterior bladder repair Is a procedure that releases the anterior vaginal wall from the bladder, folds the supportive tissue, and secures it to tighten the vaginal wall and repair urethroceles or cystoceles. Different techniques are employed, depending upon the degree of prolapse. This procedure is not specifically done for control of urinary incontinence, but repairing the prolapse may resolve the incontinence.

Surgical procedure involves either a general or spinal anesthesia. The procedure is performed through a vaginal incision. Usually a Foley catheter is inserted into the bladder and left for the first day or two until the swelling recedes. Then, urination about every 2 hours is needed to prevent pressure on the bladder. A liquid diet is followed by a low residue diet when normal bowel function occurs. Stool softeners or laxatives are used to prevent constipation. The "knack" maneuver should be done when coughing, sneezing, or doing activities that induce abdominal stress.

NEEDLE SUSPENSION

Needle suspension places stitches through the pubic skin or an incision on both sides of the bladder neck and attaches them to muscle tissue or the pubic bone for support. Surgery may be done with general or spinal anesthetic.

- The **Stamey procedure** is done vaginally or suprapubically with nylon sutures suspending the urethra.
- The **Raz procedure** uses a vaginal incision and releases fibroid bands around the bladder neck and urethra. Suspending sutures lift the anterior vagina and urethra.
- The **Gittes procedure** is done suprapubically through a small puncture. A needle is inserted through the puncture and the vaginal wall and then the suture is pulled back through the opening and secured with another suture, suspending the anterior vagina. A second puncture and suspending suture is placed about 2 cm from the first site.

A Foley catheter is usually in place for about 10 days after surgery. Difficulty urinating may result from overcorrection.

INJECTABLE BULKING IMPLANTS

Injectable bulking implants include collagen or silicone injected into the tissue about the urethra, increasing bulk of the surrounding tissue and compressing the urethra. This procedure, for both men and women, is done through a cystoscope with regional, general, or local anesthetic. The bulking material is injected through the cystoscope or, in some cases, into the skin around the sphincter. The procedure usually takes only 20-40 minutes and may be done as an outpatient. Often 2 or 3 additional implants need to be done to achieve continence. There may be urinary retention postoperative, but it is generally transient. Usually clean intermittent catheterization is done for a few days after the treatment until swelling recedes. There is usually initial improvement followed a relapse of incontinence about a week or so later and then gradual improvement again. It takes about 1 month to determine the effectiveness of the procedure.

RETROPUBIC COLPOSUSPENSION

Retropubic colposuspension lifts the bladder neck and urethra by attaching bladder and urethra or the vaginal wall to other pelvic structures**.** Surgery is done under general or spinal anesthetic with an open suprapubic incision or through laparoscopy. The **Burch procedure** is most common and requires a wide abdominal incision. The urethra and bladder neck are secured with lateral sutures through the muscles along the pubic bones. **Marshall-Marchetti-Krantz** is a similar procedure that anchors the urethra and bladder neck to cartilage; however, it poses more risk of scarring than the Burch procedure. A suprapubic catheter is left in place for about 5 days and there may be difficulty urinating initially. If this persists, corrective surgery is done to release the urethra to a more normal position. Person must refrain from strenuous activities for 3 months after surgery. Urethral kinking may occur after the Burch procedure. People have less bleeding and less pain after laparoscopy.

Percutaneous Sling Procedure

Percutaneous sling procedure uses a piece of ligament or muscle tendon, usually from the thigh or abdomen, or synthetic material to create a sling under the urethra and bladder neck to lift it to normal position. The graft is then secured to the abdominal wall and pelvic bone. The sling compresses the urethra, pushing it back into normal position. There are a number of different procedures. **Surgery** may be done under general anesthesia through a vaginal or suprapubic incision, or both. It may also be done with laparoscopy. A Foley catheter and vaginal packing are inserted during surgery and a suprapubic catheter may also be inserted. The catheters are usually removed shortly after surgery. Serious complications from this procedure are not common, but urethral obstruction can occur if the sling is too tight. If this occurs, revision may be necessary. If the sling is too loose, a suprapubic revision is usually tried.

Tension Free Vaginal Tape Procedure

Tension-free vaginal tape procedure uses a mesh-like synthetic tape under urethra to form a sling to lift it to normal position. The tape is inserted through the vagina and attached to both sides of the urethra to support the bladder neck. Within a few weeks, tissue forms about the tape and holds it in place.

Surgery is done with a local anesthesia and conscious sedation. Usually a small incision is made in the vagina, and occasionally in the suprapubic area, depending upon the procedure used. Once the tape is in place, the person is asked to cough to test the tape's support of the urethra. The procedure takes only about 30 minutes and causes only mild pain. A Foley catheter or intermittent catheterization may be used temporarily. The person is asked not to drive for 2 weeks and to avoid sexual intercourse or strenuous activities, such as sports, for 6 weeks.

Bowel Dysfunction and Fecal Incontinence Management

Management Strategies for Constipation and Fecal Impaction

Management strategies for constipation and impaction include:

- **Add fiber** with bran, fresh/dried fruits, and whole grains, to 20-35 grams per day.
- **Increase fluids** to 64 ounces each day.
- **Exercise** program should include walking if possible, and exercises on a daily basis.
- **Change in medications** causing constipation can relieve constipation. Additionally, use of stool softeners, such as Colace, or bulk formers, such as Metamucil, may decrease fluid absorption and move stool through the colon more quickly. Overuse of laxatives can cause constipation.
- **Irritable bowel syndrome** requires careful monitoring of diet, fluids and medical treatment.
- **Pregnancy-related** constipation may be controlled through dietary and fluid modifications and regular exercise.
- **Delayed toileting** should be avoided and bowel training regimen done to promote evacuation at the same time each day. During travel, stool softeners, increased fluid, and exercise may alleviate constipation.
- Enemas and manual removal of impaction may be necessary initially.

Removal of Fecal Impaction

The procedure for removal of fecal impaction is explained below:

- Gather equipment and supplies.
- Position person on left side in bed with plastic bed protection, or sitting on the toilet and leaning forward onto a pillow-covered stool or chair.
- Insert lubricated gloved finger into rectum, gently encircling mass to assess size and hardness.
- Administer oil retention enema to soften stool, guiding nozzle to side of mass. Encourage person to breathe deeply and walk about or move from side to side, while retaining enema for 30 minutes, if possible.
- Break up impaction after oil has passed or after 30-60 minutes if oil retained. Gently break up and remove stool, pulling pieces through the rectum.
- Encourage evacuation without undue straining.
- Enema, usually soapsuds, should follow even if rectal vault empty because stool may be impacted higher.
- Laxative and/or stool softener may be needed.
- Institute bowel training with diet and fluid modifications as needed.

Management of Diarrhea

Management of diarrhea includes the following:

- Institute dietary modification includes limiting alcohol and caffeine, which can cause loose stools. Artificial sugar substitutes, such as sorbitol and mannitol, should be avoided. People with lactose intolerance should use Lactaid with dairy products. Yogurt helps control diarrhea from antibiotic use. Increase foods that thicken stool, such as bananas, and soluble fiber.
- Rule-out bacterial, viral, and parasitic infections and treat as needed.

- Avoid foods or additives that trigger diarrhea.
- Stop medications that are causing diarrhea. Antibiotics frequently cause diarrhea.
- Restore fluid and electrolyte imbalance through diet, adequate fluids, or supplements, Gatorade.
- Use antidiarrheals including anti-motilities, such as Lomotil (diphenoxylate and atropine) and loperamide; Bismuth compounds, such as Pepto-Bismol; and absorbents may be used to get diarrhea under control.
- Treat underlying disease process, such as inflammatory bowel disease or Crohn's disease.
- Treat laxative abuse resulting in cycle of constipation and diarrhea.

Secca Procedure for Control of Fecal Incontinence

The Secca procedure is done as a non-surgical procedure, on an outpatient basis with conscious sedation and a local pudendal and perianal nerve block. It takes only about 45 minutes. It involves using radiofrequency energy delivered by a small generator to a hand piece with one end that is inserted into the anal canal. When triggered, small needle electrodes pierce the mucosa and radiofrequency energy causes small thermal lesions that result in shrinkage of the tissue and tightening of the anal sphincters as collagen deposits and the tissue begins to contract about the lesions. It may take several months for complete healing, but it improves fecal continence and perception of the urge to defecate in most people. This procedure is used if conservative treatment is ineffective or if sphincter repair fails. There is little pain involved with the procedure and complications are rare. Studies have shown about a 70% decrease in fecal incontinence after 6 months.

Procedure for Sacral Nerve Stimulation for Fecal Incontinence

Sacral nerve stimulation **(sacral neuromodulation)** involves stimulating the nerves that travel from the spine to enervate the rectum and anal sphincters. It is useful when there are functional defects but not structural ones. This procedure assists with neurological control of the sphincter. Nerve evaluation is done percutaneously with temporary electrodes places in the lower spine with an external stimulator for about two weeks to make sure that the nerves are intact and there is adequate response of the pelvic floor muscles. If this is successful, a permanent electrode is implanted and attached to a neurostimulator in the lower abdomen. The electrical impulse can be adjusted post-surgically by use of an external programmer. The implanted neurotransmitter lasts 5-10 years after which it needs to be replaced. This procedure has been especially helpful for those with spinal cord trauma and those with urge fecal incontinence. This treatment is less invasive than other surgical treatments.

Medications and Treatments for Fecal Incontinence

The following are medications for fecal incontinence:

- **Antidiarrheals**: to decrease diarrhea, increase tone of rectal muscle, decrease fluid content, and protect the lining of the intestine from irritation.
- **Cholinergic medications**: Decrease intestinal motility and secretions.
- **Opium derivatives**: Increase intestinal muscle tone and decrease motility.
- **Laxatives**: Treat constipation, useful with neurological deficits.
- **Stool softeners**: Increase fluid in stool.
- **Rectal stimulants**: Increase contractions to evacuate stool.
- **Hormones**: For post-menopausal women.

Additional **treatment** consists of the following:

- Diet:
  - High fiber products: Absorb fluid/add bulk. Add slowly to diet.
  - Food allergies or intolerances: need evaluation. Removing items from diet and reintroducing one at a time helps identify foods to avoid.
- Bowel training: Combines medication/diet/enemas for evacuation. It is useful for neurological deficits.
- Biofeedback: Trains people to respond to rectal distention by contracting pelvic floor and external sphincter muscles.
- Procon incontinence device: Catheter with sensor inserted into rectum with inflatable balloon to prevent leakage.

Containment Devices for Fecal Incontinence and Preventive Skin Care

Absorbent pads, briefs, disposable underwear used for fecal incontinence are the same products used for urinary leakage. Briefs usually can be refastened and often have a plastic liner on the outside, giving added protection but are noisier and bulkier than disposable underwear, which pull on like panties or shorts. Refastenable briefs are useful for the person who is bed bound or not independent in care.

The **anal bag** protects the anus and perianal area from contamination and irritation caused by fecal incontinence. It is a plastic pouch that attaches around the anus with adhesive for a secure fit and is removed and disposed of as needed.

Preventive skin care includes scrupulous hygiene, washing the soiled area with water or disposable wipes, drying thoroughly, and applying a skin barrier cream, such as Desitin or A & D ointment as needed. Soiled containment devices should be removed as soon as possible to prevent skin irritation.

Indwelling Fecal Diversion System

Indwelling fecal diversion systems are used for incontinent clients with loose or watery stools in order to prevent skin breakdown, discomfort, odor, and contamination of wounds, and to control the spread of organisms, such as *Clostridioides difficile,* in bedridden or immobile clients. A number of different devices, such as the Flexi-Seal FMS, are available and work similarly. A typical management system includes:

- silicone catheter
- silicone retention balloon at end of catheter
- 45-mL syringe
- lubricant
- charcoal filter collection bags.

The application of the fecal management system (FMS)is relatively simple: The balloon portion of the catheter is lubricated and the catheter is inserted into the rectum and balloon inflated with water or saline (using the 45 mL syringe) to hold it in place and to block fecal leakage. Some systems, such as Flexi-Seal FMS, have a pop-up button to indicate when the balloon is adequately filled for the size of the rectum. The catheter contains an irrigation port so that irrigating fluid can be instilled if necessary. The charcoal filter collection bag is attached to the end of the silicone catheter to contain fecal material.

Bowel Retraining

Bowel retraining is a behavioral modification program that helps people establish control over bowel disorders. It teaches strategies to develop a routine schedule for defecation.

- The person keeps a bowel diary for a week.
- Diet and fluid intake are modified to assure normal stool consistency. This may include increased fiber and fluids, eating meals at scheduled times, and avoiding foods that increase bowel dysfunction.
- A schedule for defecation is established, preferably at the same time each day and about 20-30 minutes after a meal, which stimulates the gastrocolic reflex that propels fecal material through the colon.
- The person is taught Kegel exercises to strengthen muscles.
- A stimulus is used to promote defecation. This may be enemas, suppositories, or laxatives in the beginning, but the goal is to decrease such use. Digital stimulation or hot drinks may be used.
- The person keeps a record of stool consistency and evacuation.

Exercise as Part of a Bowel Program

Exercise increases the motility of the bowel by stimulating muscle contractions. Walking is one of the best exercises for this purpose, and the person should try to walk one or two miles a day. If the person is unable to walk, then other activities, such as chair exercises that involve the arms and legs and bending can be very effective. Those who are bed bound need to turn from side to side frequently and change position.

Kegel exercises increase strength of the pelvic floor muscles. Kegel exercises for urinary incontinence and fecal incontinence are essentially the same, but the person tries to pull in the muscles around the anus, as though trying to prevent the release of stool or flatus. The person should feel the muscles tightening while holding for 2 seconds and then relaxing for 2, gradually building the time holding time to 10 seconds or more. Exercises should be done 4 times a day.

Suppositories

Suppositories are used to stimulate defecation for those with spinal injuries or with normal stools but tight sphincter.

1. Insert suppository rectally, guiding with gloved finger high into the rectum to the side of the rectal wall rather than in the middle of stool.
2. Sit on toilet or commode as sitting allows gravity to bring stool down.
3. Massage abdomen along the colon, from lower right abdomen, up to ribs, across abdomen, and down left side. Repeat the sequence about 10 times with 30 seconds rest in between for a total of 5-10 minutes.
4. Wait 10-15 minutes for bowel movement.
5. If no bowel movement after 15 minutes, digitally stimulate rectum. Insert lubricated gloved finger 2-3 inches inside the anus, moving finger around the walls of the rectum to stimulate the inner sphincter.
6. After evacuation, repeat digital stimulation 2 or 3 times with 5-10 minutes wait time between to ensure empty bowel.

Laxatives

Stimulants

Stimulants increase intestinal motility, moving the stool through the bowel faster and reducing the absorption of fluids so that the stool remains softer. Common ingredients include cascara in Castor oil, senna in Senokot and sennosides in Ex-lax. Stimulants work quickly and are effective but can result in electrolyte imbalance, Abdominal distension, and cramping. Chronic use may cause a cycle of constipation and diarrhea. Stimulant suppositories, such as Dulcolax are also available. Lubiprostone, marketed as Amitiza (by prescription) taken twice daily increases chloride, sodium, and water secretion from the intestinal lining, and is a treatment that softens stools and increases frequency of defecation. The FDA approved the drug in February 2006 for treatment of chronic idiopathic constipation. Prucalopride (Motegrity) enhances colonic peristalsis to promote bowel motility and was approved by the FDA for the treatment of chronic idiopathic constipation in 2018. Plecanatide (Trulance) once daily was approved in 2017 to treat the same condition by stimulating the upper GI tract to secrete fluids to support bowel function.

Bulk Formers, Lubricants, and Saline

Bulk formers have high fiber content and both soften stool and create more formed stools. These include products such as Metamucil, Citrucel, and FiberCon, which are usually added to liquids because without adequate fluids, they can increase constipation.

Lubricants include both oral mineral oil and glycerin suppositories. They coat the stool, preventing fluid absorption and keeping the stool soft. Mineral oil absorbs fat soluble vitamins and should be used only temporarily

Saline, such as Milk of Magnesia and Epsom Salt, contain ions, such as magnesium phosphate, magnesium hydroxide, and citrate, which are not absorbed through the intestines and draw more fluid into the stool. The magnesium in the preparations also stimulates the bowel. People with impairment of kidney function should avoid magnesium products, and saline laxatives should be used infrequently to avoid dependence. Epsom Salt often has a purging effect and is rarely used.

Stool Softeners, Hyperosmotics, and Combination

Stool softeners (emollients) such as Colace, and Phillip's Liqui-Gels use wetting agents, such as docusate sodium, to increase liquid in the stool, thereby softening it. They should not be used with mineral oil because of increased absorption of the oil through the intestines.

Hyperosmotics (available by prescription) contain materials that are not digestible and serve to retain fluid in the stool. Products, such as Kristalose and MiraLAX soften the stool but may result in increased Abdominal distension and flatus, especially initially. There are 3 types of hyperosmolar laxatives: lactulose, polymer, and saline. Lactulose types use a form of sugar and work similarly to saline laxatives, but more slowly, and may be used for long-term treatment. The salines empty the bowels quickly and are used short-term. The polymers contain polyethylene glycol, which retains fluid in the stool and is used short-term.

Combinations use two or more types, such as stool softener with stimulant and should be used only short-term.

Enemas

The following are different types of enemas:

- **Medicated retention** enemas may contain antibiotics, nutritives, or anti-helminthics.
- **Oil retention** enemas use mineral oil to coat and soften stool in the rectum. Usually 3-8 ounces is used. Oil retention enemas come prepackaged in single use bulb-type devices. This enema is mild and often used for children who require enemas. It is also useful as the first step in removal of an impaction because it lubricates the stool.
- **Tap water** (hypotonic) enemas are used for mechanical flushing of the rectum, but tap water if used consistently can deplete electrolytes as well as causing acute water intoxication, especially in children and the elderly, if water is retained. However, the risk if very slight if small volumes of water, which do not overwhelm the system, are used. Volume is usually 500-1000 mL, and they are effective in 15-20 minutes.

Surgical Treatments for Fecal Incontinence

Surgical options for the treatment of fecal incontinence include:

- **Rectal sphincteroplasty** involves a curved incision around the anus, loosening the sphincter muscle and then cutting away weak or damaged muscle from the anal sphincter. The remaining muscle is overlapped and reattached in order to strengthen the sphincter. The bowel is cleansed preoperatively and diet restricted to prevent passage of stool to protect the incision from infection immediately postoperatively. Constipation and hard stools might damage the surgical repair, so tool softeners or laxatives may be used initially. Activities that could strain the surgical site, such as sports or sexual activity, need to be avoided for 2-3 months.
- **Gracilis muscle transplant** uses muscle usually removed from inner thigh and transplanted to circle the rectal sphincter and provide muscle tone to compensate for loss of nerve function. Postoperative repair is similar to that of sphincteroplasty.
- **Colostomy/ileostomy for fecal diversion** involves removing all or part of the colon and diverting stool to a stoma in the abdominal wall.

Artificial Anal Sphincter

The artificial anal sphincter consists of an inflatable cuff surgically implanted around the anal sphincter to prevent fecal leakage, a reservoir in the lower abdomen, and a pump with a button to push usually in the labia of females or scrotum of males. The artificial sphincter is used for intractable fecal incontinence. The procedure is usually done with a general or a spinal anesthesia after cleansing bowel preparation. There are different pressure settings available for the cuffs. Following surgery, the cuff is usually not inflated for about 6-8 weeks while the tissue is healing. The cuff is deflated when a person wants to have a bowel movement, and it automatically reinflates in about 10 minutes. Activities that apply pressure to the rectal area, such as bicycle riding, may cause trauma and irritation. Infection can occur because of fecal contamination of the tissues, and mechanical failure can necessitate removal or replacement of the device.

Continent Appendicostomy (Malone Continence Enema [MACE] Procedure)

Continent appendicostomy (Malone continence enema [MACE] procedure) is frequently used with children who suffer neuromuscular impairment, resulting from congenital disorders (myelomeningocele), anorectal malformations, spinal injuries, and Hirschsprung's disease. It can also be used for adults with intractable constipation. In this procedure, the appendix or part of the cecum is brought to abdominal wall to form a stoma, usually at the umbilicus, to provide an open channel into the ascending colon for insertion of a catheter to provide antegrade irrigation. The

Malone procedure may be done with and open procedure or a laparoscopy. A catheter is placed through the channel during surgery and left in place for about 3 weeks to allow healing. An antegrade enema is usually given about the 2nd day postoperatively and then every 2-3 days or as needed to control evacuation. Successful control of fecal incontinence is about 90% with this procedure.

MACE Irrigations

MACE irrigations are usually done with tap water, although normal saline may be used, about 900 mL average for an adult, but ranging from 500 mL to 2000 mL. For children 50 mL is used initially and then the amount is increased gradually with each irrigation, until optimum results are achieved. Sometimes, people are advised to add a small amount of mineral oil or Fleet's enema:

- Gather supplies and equipment
- Insert latex free straight or Foley catheter with 5 mL balloon (usually 12-14 Fr.) into stoma to prescribed distance. Inflate balloon if using Foley. Using a Foley catheter frees both hands as the balloon holds the catheter in place.
- Attach enema bag and tubing and slowly instill solution.
- Clamp tube.
- Deflate Foley/remove catheter.
- Cleanse equipment and wash catheter, which should be replaced every 2-3 weeks.

Dietary Management of Bowel Dysfunction

Dietary management requires identifying foods that increase bowel dysfunction by keeping a list of foods for a week to correlate with bowel activity. **Foods** to avoid include spicy, cured, or smoked meats and fatty and greasy foods that often cause diarrhea and fecal incontinence. Lactose intolerants should avoid dairy products. Caffeine, alcohol, and artificial sweeteners, such as aspartame, NutraSweet, and saccharine can act as laxatives so they and foods that contain them, like sugar-free gum and diet soda, should be avoided, although Splenda and stevia are usually acceptable.

- **Several small meals** instead of large meals may reduce bowel contractions.
- **Fiber** increased to 20-30 grams per day makes stool formed and easier to control although too much can cause bloating and gas, so it's important to add fiber slowly to the diet. Eating whole fruits, whole grains, and vegetables increases fiber.
- **Fluid intake** should be at least 8 glasses, especially water, daily to prevent constipation and impaction.

Fiber in the Diet

Most constipation is caused by insufficient fiber in the diet, especially if people eat a lot of processed foods. An adequate amount of fiber is 20-30 grams daily. There are both soluble and insoluble forms of fiber, and both add bulk to the stool and are not absorbed into the body. Some foods have both types:

- **Soluble fiber** dissolves in liquids to form a gel-like substance, one reason why liquids are so important in conjunction with fiber in the diet. Soluble fiber slows the movement of stool through the gastrointestinal system. Food sources include bananas, starches (potatoes, bread), cheese, dried beans, nuts apples, oranges, and oatmeal.
- **Insoluble fiber** changes little with the digestive process and increases the speed of stool through the colon, so too much can result in diarrhea. Food sources of insoluble fiber include oat bran, seeds, skins of fruits and vegetables and nuts.

Increasing Fiber in the Diet and Promoting Optimum Bowel Health

Establishing a regular routine of eating certain types of foods easiest does increasing fiber. Foods that are high in fiber are often also rich sources of nutrients:

- Start the day with bran cereal, or add 1-2 Tablespoons bran to other foods.
- Substitute whole or dried fruit (including the skin when possible) for juice.
- Eat whole grain breads instead of white bread.
- Eat vegetables, such as broccoli, or dried beans.
- Eat a handful of nuts each day.
- Eat a big salad at least once a day.

Changing how a person eats can also help maintain good bowel function:

- Instead of 3 big meals, eat 5 or 6 small meals.
- Drink at least 8 glasses of liquid a day and drink before meals to help absorb soluble fiber.
- Avoid foods and drinks that trigger diarrhea or constipation

Continence Care: Education and Referral

Patient and Health Care Professional Education

Patient Education for Wound Management

Patients should be educated on the following elements of wound management:

- **Infection control**: Topics include the importance of hand hygiene, methods for disposal of soiled materials, the risk of healthcare-associated infections (including asking healthcare providers to wash hands), appropriate use of antibiotics, and appropriate wound care.
- **Repositioning**: The need for repositioning, the manner, positions, and frequency vary depending on the patient's condition, but the patient should be apprised of the importance of repositioning to prevent skin breakdown and shown how to reposition, encouraging the patient to reposition at least every 2 hours.
- **Trauma avoidance**: Topics include fall prevention and safe driving as well as measures to improve home safety, such as removal of throw rugs and clutter, improved lighting, installation of handrails and safety bars, and use of shower chairs. Some patients may need information about avoiding choking, fire safety, and safe use of tools (such as knives and clippers)

Tobacco Cessation

Smoking releases carbon monoxide and hydrogen cyanide in the blood and interferes with the delivery of oxygen to the tissues, and nicotine is a vasoconstrictor, resulting in slowed healing. Smoking also increases platelet clumping, increasing risk of clotting. Patients should learn about the effects of smoking on healing and should be provided tobacco cessation aids. A number of medical treatments can assist patients through the withdrawal period, during which the person may experience anxiety, irritability, and nicotine craving. Many of the of the medications contain nicotine, but it is released in a slower manner to avoid the sudden increase in nicotine ("rush") associated with smoking: Nicotine patch, nicotine inhaler, nicotine gum, nicotine lozenge, and nicotine nasal spray. Prescription medications that are taken before quitting and then for up to 6 months include bupropion SR and varenicline. Smoking cessation programs include support groups, online forums (StopSmokingCenter.net) and informational websites (Smokefree.gov). The HHS recommends the 5A program: Ask, advise, assess, assist, and arrange followup.

Behavioral Strategies

Dietary Management to Control Urinary Incontinence

Dietary management of urinary incontinence requires some modifications.

- **Foods** that are bladder irritants, such as spicy foods, citrus fruits, and tomatoes should be avoided altogether or rarely eaten. Most sugar substitutes should be avoided although Splenda and stevia may be used.
- **Fluid intake** may be limited to less than the optimal 60 ounces per day although too much restriction can result in dehydration and constipation, further aggravating the incontinence. A good plan is to spread intake out through the day and restrict fluids in the evening, especially if nocturia or enuresis is a problem. Alcohol, which has a diuretic effect, should be avoided or used only occasionally. Apple juice or grape juice can be substituted for orange juice or cranberry juice as they are less irritating to the bladder. De-caffeinated tea and coffee should be used or coffee limited to one cup per day. Carbonated drinks, most of which contain caffeine should be avoided.

Behavioral Techniques for Treatment of Urinary Incontinence

Behavioral techniques for treating urinary incontinence include:

- **Biofeedback**: Training to control bladder and sphincter muscles.
- **Bladder training**: Training to lengthen time between urination: may include double voiding to make sure bladder empties completely. Relaxation techniques are used to control urge to urinate. Timed urination, scheduled usually every 2-4 hours, helps to prevent incontinence.
- **Diet**: Avoid foods that irritate the bladder, such as acidic foods. Alcohol and caffeine intake may need to be limited. Monitoring fluid intake and reducing fluids in the evening are often helpful.
- **Electrical stimulation**: Pelvic floor muscles are stimulated by the temporary insertion of electrodes into the rectum or vagina. Because it can take months for treatment to be effective, and there are many side effects, it is often used only for those who haven't responded to other treatments and have severe incontinence.
- **Kegel (pelvic floor) exercises**: Strengthen the pelvic floor muscles and the urinary sphincter. They are usually done 3-4 times daily, for stress incontinence.

Pelvic Muscle Exercises and Methods to Isolate Pelvic Floor Muscles

Pelvic muscle exercises, also known as Kegel exercises, are used to strengthen the periurethral and pelvic muscles in order to increase control of urination and fecal incontinence. Basic exercises involve tightening the muscles 3-4 times daily for about 3 seconds and then relaxing for the same period, repeating about 10 times and gradually increasing the time tightening the muscles to 5-10 seconds.

Isolating the right muscles to tighten is important. Tightening the stomach, leg, or other muscles will not help. People should not hold their breath during the exercises because this may tighten other muscles. There are three methods to check that the pelvic floor muscles are flexing:

1. Stop flow of urine in the midst of urination.
2. Pull in the anus as though trying to stop from passing flatus.
3. In supine position, place finger inside the vagina and squeeze as though trying to stop urine. Tightness should be felt.

Positions for Pelvic Floor Muscle Exercises

Pelvic floor muscle exercises can be done anywhere, such as at work or while sitting in a restaurant, as they will not be obvious to others. It's important that people establish a schedule for exercises and try to maintain the schedule, even if not at home. These exercises can be done in different positions:

- **Sitting** exercises are done in a straight-back chair with a firm seat and with feet planted on the floor or legs stretched out and ankles crossed.
- **Reclining** exercises are done lying flat with head on a pillow and knees bent, with feet apart slightly. Knees may be supported with a pillow to prevent tightening of thigh muscles.
- **Standing** exercises are done while holding onto a surface, such as a chair or counter, for support. Knees should be bent slightly with feet about 1 foot apart. Alternately, one can lean against a counter with hips flexed.

PFES

Pelvic floor electrical stimulation (PFES) is the application of low-grade electrical stimulation to the pelvic floor muscles to provide a passive contraction, stimulating the pelvic muscles to contract. It is used to rehabilitate weakened muscles. PFES of the pudendal nerve causes a pudendal nerve reflex loop that results in muscle contraction. PFES is used to assist with isolating the pelvic floor muscles for those who have not been successful with Kegel exercises. It increases the strength of pelvic muscle contraction, it decreases ineffective and uninhibited contraction of the detrusor muscle, and it helps to normalize pelvic muscle relaxation. PFES is applied with skin electrodes around the anus or with vaginal or rectal sensor probes. PFES is often done in conjunction with biofeedback because PFES makes the person more aware of pelvic floor muscle activity and biofeedback helps the person to gain control of the bladder by using these muscles.

Components

Key components of PFES units:

- **Waveform** is shape of the impulse on a graph. The waveform for muscle stimulation is rectangular, bi-phasic, and bipolar, a type not damaging to tissue.
- **Amplitude** is strength and intensity of current, which must be enough to create an "anal wink."
- **Ramping** is the speed with which the current reaches the muscles. The faster the current rises, the more discomfort is felt.
- **Frequency rate** is the number of pulses or hertz (Hz) per second. The frequency rate for stress incontinence is 50 Hz, which builds muscle and tightens urethral sphincters; for urge incontinence, 13 Hz, which calms the detrusor muscle and prevents bladder contractions.
- **On/off time** is the ratio of time the muscle is exposed to electrical current and time the muscle recovers. Time on must be less than time off. A typical ratio is 1:2, such as on 5 seconds and off 10.

Pharmacological Treatments for Urinary Incontinence

Pharmacological treatments are those oral and topical medications that have helped control urinary incontinence:

- **Adrenergic agents**, such as or Sudafed, increase pressure on urethra and prevent stress incontinence.
- **Antibiotics**, such as Bactrim, treat urinary infections that exacerbate incontinence.
- **Anticholinergics**, such as oxybutynin and tolterodine serve to relax detrusor and pelvic floor muscles and reduce frequency. They may also increase bladder capacity and are useful for overactive bladder because they block the chemicals that stimulate bladder nerves.
- **Estrogens**, such as Premarin (oral) and Estrace (topical) improve muscles tone and prevent atrophic changes of the mucosa.
- **Serotonin norepinephrine reuptake inhibitor** duloxetine (Cymbalta) increases urethral sphincter contraction during storage phase.
- **Smooth muscle relaxants** to relieve bladder spasms.
- **Tricyclic antidepressants**, such as imipramine, increase urinary sphincter tone and decrease bladder spasms.
- **Urinary analgesics**, such as phenazopyridine, alleviate spasms and discomfort caused by urinary infections.

Voiding Diaries

Bladder Diary

Bladder diary is a complete daily record of all urinations and episodes of urinary incontinence. The diary is usually kept for 3-5 days as part of the urological assessment and includes the following:

- **Time** must be recorded to document patterns of urination.
- **Amount** of urination should be estimated (small, medium, or large) or measured as directed.
- **Intake** should be recorded to determine if fluids are contributing to incontinence or urinary problems.
- **Incontinence** should be characterized by estimations of amount. A small volume of less than 30 mL is enough to wet underwear. A moderate volume of 30-60 mL is enough to soak underwear with overflow down legs. A large volume of more than 60 mL is usually enough to soak clothes and run onto floor or furniture.
- **Incontinence** should be characterized by activity and sensation of urge at time of incontinence to help determine the type of incontinence.

Bowel Diary

Bowel diary is a complete daily record of all defecations and episodes of fecal or flatal incontinence. The diary is usually kept for 3-5 days as part of the intestinal assessment and includes the following:

- **Time** of each event should be carefully documented.
- **Type** of bowel movement should be noted, using the Bristol Stool Form Scale or other guide: hard lumps, sausage-shaped, cracked sausage-shaped, smooth and snake-like, soft blobs, fluffy pieces, or liquid.
- **Amount** of stool should be estimated.
- **Abnormalities** such as blood or mucous and the need for finger splinting or straining should be noted.
- **Fecal incontinence** should be characterized by amount and type and activity at the time of incontinence.
- **Flatal incontinence** should be noted.
- **Intake** of both food and fluids should be recorded to see if intake relates to bowel activities.
- **Medications** should all be recorded, including laxatives, vitamins, and any over-the-counter preparations.

Emptying Maneuver to Control Urinary Incontinence

Trigger Voiding

Trigger voiding is a technique that is useful for those with spinal cord injuries or neurogenic bladders. It involves finding the "trigger" that initiates contraction of the bladder. One method is **suprapubic tapping**, in which the person drums the fingers over the bladder area, above the pubic bone. Usually the suprapubic area is tapped 7 or 8 times, followed by a rest period of 3 seconds, and then the tapping is repeated. The rhythmic tapping is believed to produce an effect on the tension receptors in the bladder wall, activating the reflex arc that results in contraction of the bladder. Trigger mechanisms may vary from one individual to another, so some trial and error is involved. Other common triggers are pulling pubic hairs, stroking the inner thighs or abdomen, digital anal stimulation and dilation, listening to running water, placing hands in warm water, pouring warm water over perineum, or drinking warm fluids.

Credé Maneuver

Credé maneuver uses direct compression over the bladder area to prompt contraction of the detrusor muscle or to complete emptying of the bladder. The technique involves applying manual pressure above the pubic bone. Pressure should be firm and even, not abrupt, and begin with a slight upward pressure followed by downward pressure. Pressure should be maintained while the bladder empties but stopped immediately if pain occurs. The Credé maneuver should not be used if the bladder is grossly distended. The Credé maneuver is usually used in conjunction with a scheduled voiding program for chronic urinary incontinence.

Double Voiding

Double voiding is a technique used with mild to moderate urinary retention. The person urinates, attempting to empty the bladder, and then stays on the toilet for 2-10 minutes and tries to urinate again. Alternately, after the initial urination, the person may stand for a brief period, sit back down, and then urinate for the second time.

Skin Care to Prevent Irritation from Fecal or Urinary Incontinence

Cleanse skin with water after each episode of incontinence. Soap tends to be drying and can cause irritation, but if soap is needed, people can use baby wash, which is quite mild, or disposable pre-moistened alcohol-free, perfume-free wipes. After cleansing, the area should be dried thoroughly, patting dry or using a hair dryer on low heat.

Apply cream or powder if there is any sign of skin irritation. Moisture-barrier creams, such as Desitin and A & D ointment can prevent urine or feces from directly contacting skin. Non-medicated, non-perfumed talcum powder or cornstarch may help to keep perineal area dry.

Wear loose clothing to allow for airflow as tight clothes can make skin irritation worse. Many synthetic fibers, such as polyester, constrict air and should be avoided. Underwear should be 100% cotton.

Incontinence pads should contain an absorbent wicking layer to keep moisture away from the skin and should be changed promptly when soiled.

Educating Health Care Providers on Incontinence Care Principles

The continence care nurse's role in educating health care providers on **incontinence care** principles includes mentoring, role modeling, and providing information:

- Explaining the different types and causes of both fecal and urinary incontinence.
- Identifying signs of incontinence and asking pertinent questions about a history of incontinence and urinary tract infections.
- Assessing factors that may contribute to incontinence, including a discussion of dietary and fluid intake and review of medications.
- Developing a personalized plan of care and toileting program as appropriate for each patient with individualized goals based on multiple factors, including type of incontinence, cognition, barriers, mobility, dependence, medications, and resources.
- Assessing potential barriers to implementation of the plan (lighting, inaccessible bathroom, analgesics, cognitive impairments) and developing compensatory measures.
- Developing and education plan for both the patient and appropriate caregivers in preparation for discharge or transfer.
- Determining appropriate methods for evaluating the effectiveness of the care plan and carrying out ongoing monitoring of patient.

Multidisciplinary Collaboration

Resources for Patients

Resources available to the patient include:

- **Support and advocacy**: Support groups are available through many medical centers and hospitals as well as online. Many are sponsored by national organizations and are generally free of cost and available to patients and/or families. National organizations also often provide information about clinical trials and current research.
- **Access to supplies**: Many manufacturers provides assistance programs for those unable to afford supplies, such as dressings, and some national organizations may also provide assistance. Some patients may be eligible for Medicaid, which will cover the costs of necessary supplies and equipment.
- **Post-acute care**: This level of care is less intense than that provided by an acute hospital. Post-acute care may be provided after acute hospitalization or instead of acute hospitalization. Medical treatments can be continued with post-acute care but the focus is more commonly on rehabilitation.

Community and National Organizations to Assist Those Managing Urinary Incontinence

There are a number of community and national organizations that can provide information and support to those who have urinary incontinence. Many of the sites listed below provide printable information sheets, lists of urologists, pictures and diagrams, information about clinical trials, newsletters, message boards, and print material, such as booklets. They are invaluable resources for persons and caregivers dealing with incontinence or other urinary conditions.

- National Institute on Aging Information Center
- National Association for Continence
- Simon Foundation for Continence
- National Institute of Diabetes and Digestive and Kidney Diseases
- American Urological Association/Urology Health.org

Resources for Patients Suffering from Functional Incontinence

Functional incontinence is incontinence that is due to physical or mental disabilities that prevent a person from being able to get to the bathroom.

- **Physical Therapy**: This service can help to individualize an exercise program that can help patients to strengthen the muscles of their pelvic floor. If there are physical mobility issues limiting a person's ability to use the bathroom, they can help with strengthening and increasing the ROM of the muscles necessary.
- **Occupational Therapy**: This can help with improving the patient's ability to perform their activities of daily living. Training can be given in transferring to the toilet, evaluating for a raised toilet seat or grab bars that could help a person in transferring, improving trunk mobility and balance, and cognitive and sequencing skills.
- **Social Worker**: This can help to address some of the psychosocial issues associated with incontinence. The patients may have problems with depression and anxiety due to their incontinence. They may be limiting their social contacts because of the risk of embarrassment, thus resulting in a low self-esteem.

Making Appropriate Consultations and Referrals

Referrals to Social Services or Mental Health Services

Patients often face many challenges and complex medical and emotional needs. The nurse plays an important role in identifying the appropriateness of **referrals** for specialized support:

- **Social services**: Costs of wound care products can be high, and patients may lack adequate income to pay for supplies or may have no or inadequate insurance. Some patients, especially older adults, may be unable to care for themselves without assistance or may lack transportation. Patients are often unaware of services for which they may be eligible. Social workers can assist patients to identify needs and government or community programs that can provide assistance.
- **Mental health professionals**: Depression, shame, and anxiety associated with wound care and body image issues may cause patients to refuse care, avoid assuming responsibility for care, or avoid social contacts. Patients may feel overwhelmed and hopeless and have difficulty expressing feelings. Those with cognitive decline may be confused. It's important to be alert to signs of distress, to utilize screening tools (such as PHQ-9 or GAD-7), and to refer patients to mental health professionals.

Consults

Patients with symptoms or needs that exceed the nurse's scope of practice or suggest underlying pathology may require **consultation** with an appropriate specialist:

- **Gastroenterology**: GI specialist may help to manage underlying disease, adjust medications, and carry out diagnostic procedures, such as endoscopy. Indications include high output ostomies, persistent diarrhea, failure of fistulae to close, and stomal complications, and short bowel syndrome.
- **Genitourinary**: GU specialist may carry out diagnostic procedures, such as cystoscopy, provide interventions (Botox, artificial sphincter), or place long-term SP catheters. Indications include incontinence, urinary retention, hematuria, and recurrent UTIs.
- **Oncology**: Oncologist may provide guidance regarding disease, modify treatments to aid wound healing, and initiate palliative care when appropriate. Indications include malignant wounds, fungating tumors, issues of wound healing associated with chemotherapy or radiation, and need for pain control.
- **Gynecology**: Gynecologist may may hormones, fit pessaries, carry out surgical repairs, and coordinate pelvic floor rehabilitation. Indications include rectovaginal and vesicovaginal fistulae, prolapse, incontinence, and chronic vulvar skin breakdown associated with incontinence.

Handoff/Transition of Patients with Incontinence

Hand-off/transition procedures for patients with incontinence should be documented and adequate time allowed for communication, including questions from the receiving party. Important elements that must be covered include:

- Demographic information, such as name, diagnoses, address, telephone number.
- List of medications and treatments.
- Physical impairments that may impact ability to self-care, such as vision impairment and impaired mobility.
- Type of incontinence (urinary and/or fecal).
- History of incontinence and conditions under which incontinence occurs.
- Complications, such as moisture-associated skin damage, dermatitis, ulcerations, maceration, fungal infections.
- Interventions utilized in the past and in the present to manage incontinence, and patient response.
- Supplies and/or equipment that is needed by the patient (catheter supplies, bedside commode).
- Education of patient/caregiver regarding incontinence, treatments, skin care, and precautions (signs of infection, skin deterioration), preventive measures, and response.
- Psychosocial factors that may present a barrier to incontinence care, such as cognitive impairments, poverty, lack of support system.
- Nutritional guidelines/interventions, such as limiting fluids in the evening and increasing fiber in diet.

Practice Test

Want to take this practice test in an online interactive format?
Check out the online resources page, which includes interactive practice questions and much more: **mometrix.com/resources719/cccn**

Continence Care

1. Which is the *BEST* solution for chemical trauma in the perianal and genital area from incontinence of urine and feces in an 87-year-old patient?

a. apply moisture barrier paste
b. apply solid moisture barrier
c. apply skin barrier powder
d. leave skin open to the air

2. What percentage of the fluid does the colon absorb from the stool as the stool traverses the bowel?

a. 30%
b. 40%
c. 60%
d. 90%

3. Which of the following occurs during phase I (filling/storing) of the urination process?

a. spinal nerves contract the detrusor muscles
b. spinal nerves relax internal sphincter muscles
c. neurotransmitters signal the detrusor muscles to relax
d. external sphincter muscles relax

4. With the Bristol Stool Form, which of the following stool types is described as sausage-shaped and lumpy with cracks on the surface?

a. type 1
b. type 2
c. type 3
d. type 4

5. Postinfectious irritable bowel syndrome (PI-IBS) is characterized most commonly by

a. fever.
b. altered bowel habits with chronic diarrhea.
c. constipation.
d. flu-like symptoms.

6. Which of the following is a typical a symptom associated with rectoceles?

a. chronic constipation
b. chronic diarrhea
c. pulling sensation in pelvic area
d. vaginal discharge

7. The PRIMARY cause of fecal incontinence with anorectal fistulae is

a. pain.
b. inflammation and tissue damage.
c. loss of sensation.
d. leakage of stool from fistula.

8. Which of the following disorders can result in chronic constipation and incontinence because of damage to the myelin sheath and underlying nerve fibers in the brain, eyes, and spinal cord?

a. Amyotrophic lateral sclerosis (ALS)
b. Parkinson's disease (PD)
c. Muscular dystrophy (MD)
d. Multiple sclerosis (MS)

9. The Q-tip test measures

a. strength of the pelvic floor muscles.
b. duration of bladder contractions.
c. length of urethra.
d. mobility and axis position of the urethra.

10. During the provocative stress test (urinary cough test), what position should the patient be placed in for the first part of the test?

a. supine position
b. standing with one leg on stool
c. prone
d. sitting

11. Which of the following is included on the mini-mental status exam?

a. reading text and then summarizing
b. timed reading test
c. counting backward by 7s or spelling "world" backward
d. drawing the face of a clock with 12 numbers and hands indicating a specific time

12. Which test measures the pressure of the anal sphincter muscles, degree of rectal sensation, and neural reflexes?

a. anal wink
b. bulbocavernosus reflex
c. endoanal ultrasound
d. anal manometry

13. Which of the following groups of foods should be avoided to prevent gas with a colostomy?

a. cabbage, broccoli, kale, onions, turnips, brussel sprouts, asparagus, dried beans, fish, eggs, and strong cheeses
b. applesauce, bananas, cheese, creamy peanut butter, potatoes, rice, pasta, marshmallows
c. apple juice, prune juice fresh fruit, raw vegetables, spicy foods, fried foods
d. dried fruits, fruits with skin, tree nuts, popcorn, whole corn, bean sprouts, celery, and large servings of raw fruits or vegetables

14. When patients keep a bladder diary, which description is estimated as equaling 30 to 60 mL volume of urinary incontinence?

a. slight spot of dampness in underwear
b. underwear wet
c. underwear soaked with overflow down legs
d. clothes soaked and overflow on floor or furniture

15. The patient is scheduled for anal sphincter electromyography. Which of the patient's medications should be stopped prior to the EMG?

a. stool softener
b. anticholinergic
c. antibiotic
d. warfarin

16. The normal specific gravity of urine is

a. 1.000 to 1.010.
b. 1.010 to 1.015.
c. 1.015 to 1.025.
d. 1.025 to 1.035.

17. When a person is doing a 24-hour pad test at home, which of the following is necessary?

a. sealing wet pads in plastic bags and storing
b. counting the number of pads used in a day
c. leaving the same pad in place for 24 hours
d. changing pads every 8 hours

18. Which of the following tests assess bladder capacity and pressure, including how full the bladder is when the urge to urinate is felt?

a. electromyography
b. uroflowmetry
c. pressure flow study
d. cystometry

19. A reduced Valsalva leak point pressure indicates

a. stress incontinence.
b. urge incontinence.
c. functional incontinence.
d. overflow incontinence.

20. When fitting a patient with a pessary for second-degree cystocele, which is correct?

a. the smallest possible pessary should be used
b. a finger should pass easily between the vaginal wall and the pessary
c. a finger should not be able to pass between the vaginal wall and the pessary.
d. should always begin with ring pessaries

21. Chronic pelvic pain syndrome results from

a. unknown etiology.
b. bacterial infection.
c. trauma.
d. viral infection.

22. Which of the following medical treatments is used to reduce urinary frequency and incontinence in patients with multiple sclerosis?

a. prophylactic low dose antibiotics
b. diuretics (such as furosemide)
c. anticholinergics (such as oxybutynin or tolterodine)
d. muscle relaxers (such as baclofen)

23. The average age for menopause is

a. 50.
b. 49.
c. 53.
d. 51.

24. Which of the following is the *MOST* significant factor in developing urinary incontinence?

a. obesity
b. diuretic use
c. history of human papillomavirus
d. history of oral contraceptive use

25. In a functional assessment, support from family or friends is evaluated as

a. nonfunction related.
b. psychological function.
c. sensory function.
d. social function.

26. Which environmental factor may *MOST* likely contribute to incontinence in a patient with severe rheumatoid arthritis affecting the hips, knees, and ankles?

a. bathroom is on the second floor from kitchen and living room
b. throw rugs are in place in the hall leading to bathroom
c. hallway to bathroom is not lit
d. toilet is too low

27. Which of the following is a bladder irritant?

a. watermelon
b. milk
c. artificial sweetener (aspartame, saccharine)
d. beef

28. The "knack" is

a. a method to prevent fecal incontinence.
b. a method to strengthen pelvic floor muscles.
c. a method to prevent urge incontinence.
d. a method to prevent stress incontinence.

29. The "quick flicks" method treats urinary incontinence by

a. improving contractility.
b. improving endurance.
c. improving sensory awareness.
d. reducing muscle spasms.

30. Which of the following is *MOST* important in controlling constipation?

a. taking daily stool softener
b. increasing exercise
c. increasing dietary fiber and fluids
d. taking laxatives

31. Incontinence of liquid stool and engorged hemorrhoids are *MOST* indicative of

a. constipation.
b. diarrhea.
c. fecal impaction.
d. rectal cancer.

32. Which of the following is a good source of soluble fiber?

a. oat bran
b. seeds
c. skins of fruits
d. bananas

33. When is the best time for scheduled defecation?

a. 20 to 30 minutes before a meal
b. 20 to 30 minutes after a meal
c. first thing in the morning
d. last thing at night

34. A woman with a coccygeal ulcer has occasional urinary incontinence but has no urinary infection. Which should be the *INITIAL* step in controlling her incontinence?

a. limited fluid intake
b. insertion of Foley catheter
c. anticholinergic medication (such as oxybutynin)
d. scheduled urination

35. Black tarry stools may be caused by

a. Rifadin.
b. Pepto-Bismol.
c. Kaopectate.
d. Beta-carotene.

36. With nocturnal enuresis, which medication can be taken at bedtime by a female patient to reduce urinary production?

a. oxybutynin
b. imipramine
c. desmopressin
d. tamsulosin

37. With vaginal weights, correct size is determined by

a. vaginal measurements.
b. the heaviest weight that fits comfortably.
c. the ability to hold the weight for one minute.
d. the smallest weight that doesn't fall out.

38. The treatment of choice for urge incontinence is

a. anticholinergics.
b. reducing bladder irritants.
c. surgical repair.
d. bladder training.

39. Which is the *INITIAL* treatment of choice for a male who develops bladder outlet obstruction from benign prostatic hypertrophy?

a. intermittent catheterization to empty bladder
b. transurethral prostatectomy
c. medications, such as alpha-blocker and 5-alpha reductase inhibitor
d. transurethral needle ablation

40. The treatment of choice for a male with detrusor sphincter dyssynergia is

a. insertion of urethral stent.
b. external sphincterectomy.
c. long-term catheterization.
d. urinary diversion.

41. Which of the following is recommended to manage detrusor hyperactivity with impaired contractile function (DHIC)?

a. anticholinergics
b. indwelling catheter
c. double voiding and Credé maneuver
d. urinary diversion

42. The most appropriate fecal containment product for an elderly bedridden patient with diminished level of consciousness, intact skin, and incontinence of approximately 400 mL of semi-liquid stool daily is

a. fecal pouch with skin barrier.
b. fecal containment system.
c. disposable underwear with skin barrier.
d. refastenable briefs with skin barrier.

43. A patient with mild dementia lives alone and has increasing urge incontinence, because she forgets to comply with scheduled urination. The best solution is

a. disposable underwear.
b. long-term catheterization.
c. an alarm.
d. telephone reminders.

44. A male using a penile clamp to control moderate urinary incontinence after prostatectomy should release the clamp and urinate

a. when the bladder feels full.
b. every 4 to 6 hours.
c. after each meal.
d. every 2 hours.

45. Which of the following is the *MOST* effective for a physically active woman to use during periods of strenuous exercise to prevent stress incontinence?

a. absorbent pads
b. tampon
c. urethral plug
d. valved catheter

46. The *PRIMARY* purpose of sensory motor reeducation using biofeedback for fecal incontinence is to

a. assist in contraction of anal sphincters.
b. increase sensory perception and control of the muscles of defecation.
c. assist in relaxation of external anal sphincters.
d. prevent fecal impaction.

47. Overuse of phosphate enemas to control constipation puts a person at risk for

a. hypermagnesemia and hypocalcemia.
b. hypomagnesemia and hypercalcemia.
c. hypophosphatemia and hypercalcemia.
d. hyperphosphatemia and hypocalcemia.

48. Which of the following procedures is done to expand bladder capacity?

a. augmentation cystoplasty
b. sling procedure
c. tension-free vaginal tape procedure (TVT)
d. retropubic suspension

49. For clean intermittent catheterization at home, which methods of sterilization are MOST effective after first cleaning and drying catheters?

a. boil for 5 minutes or microwave for 3 minutes on high
b. boil for 10 minutes OR microwave on high for 6 minutes with a glass of water in the microwave
c. boil for 5 to 8 minutes
d. microwave for 4 minutes on high with a glass of water in the microwave

50. During pelvic floor electrical stimulation, which serves as a guide that adequate amplitude has been set?

a. anal wink occurs
b. the patient reports muscle contractions
c. standardized setting guidelines have been used
d. the patient feels pain

51. For female patients undergoing anal sphincteroplasty, the most common problem in the postoperative period is

a. infection.
b. difficulty urinating.
c. severe pain.
d. separation of sutures.

52. The first indication that a patient may develop fecal incontinence is

a. flatus incontinence.
b. chronic constipation.
c. mucus incontinence.
d. chronic diarrhea.

53. If a patient is diagnosed with detrusor external sphincter dyssynergia (DESD), the nurse expects the treatment plan to include

a. indwelling catheter.
b. urinary diversion.
c. augmentation cystoplasty.
d. clean intermittent catheterization.

54. If a patient has quit smoking and has been chewing sugar free gum and snacking on carrots, nuts, and celery all day to control cravings, but has developed bloating and recurrent diarrhea, the most likely cause of the diarrhea is

a. sugar free chewing gum.
b. carrots.
c. nuts.
d. celery.

55. If using ultrasound scanning to decrease obsessive toileting for a patient with overactive bladder, the patient should be urged to delay urination if the bladder volume is less than

a. 50 to 75 mL.
b. 100 to 150 mL.
c. 175 to 200 mL.
d. 200 to 225 mL.

56. Patients with fecal incontinence often try to self-manage for years before discussing the problem with healthcare providers primarily because they

a. don't believe help is available.
b. don't want to bother the healthcare provider.
c. feel shame and embarrassment about the incontinence.
d. aren't concerned about the fecal incontinence.

57. The most common cause of fecal incontinence in females is

a. neurological disease.
b. obstetric trauma.
c. constipation and straining.
d. irritable bowel syndrome.

58. When treating urge urinary incontinence with pelvic floor electrical stimulation, the frequency rate, pps/Hz, should be set at

a. 13 pps.
b. 20 pps.
c. 50 pps.
d. 100 pps.

59. If a patient is undergoing bladder training and is trying to resist the urge to urinate for one-hour periods but feels a strong urge to urinate after 40 minutes, the patient should be advised to

a. urinate.
b. avoid urinating for 20 minutes.
c. avoid urinating for 1 to 3 minutes.
d. practice distraction techniques.

60. If the urinalysis is positive for leukocyte esterase, this usually indicates

a. normal finding.
b. pregnancy.
c. pyuria.
d. fungal infection.

61. Which of the following types of pessaries is MOST appropriate for treatment for cystocele and stress urinary incontinence?

a. Gehring with knob.
b. donut.
c. ring.
d. Gelhorn soft silicone with standard stem.

62. Smoking increases the risk of urinary incontinence, especially

a. urge incontinence.
b. stress incontinence.
c. overflow incontinence.
d. functional incontinence.

63. Reservoir fecal incontinence is associated with

a. anal sphincter damage.
b. constipation/fecal impaction.
c. neurological impairment.
d. decreased colonic or rectal capacity.

64. Which of the following tests is used to determine the amount of fecal material the rectum can accommodate and how effectively the stool is expelled?

a. anorectal ultrasonography
b. balloon expulsion test
c. proctography
d. anal manometry

65. For patients with fecal incontinence, the most troubling physical effect is generally

a. sensation of incomplete emptying of bowels.
b. rectal irritation.
c. cramping.
d. urgency.

66. Which of the following medications may relieve flatus incontinence?

a. psyllium fiber
b. simethicone
c. docusate sodium
d. loperamide

67. During an interview, older patients often fail to mention urinary incontinence because they

a. forget about it.
b. don't feel it is burdensome.
c. believe it is a natural part of aging.
d. successfully manage it.

68. If a patient with no previous fecal incontinence has developed a sudden onset of slow leakage of stool and a feeling of rectal discomfort, the patient should first be assessed for

a. rectal cancer.
b. fecal impaction.
c. medication-associated incontinence.
d. internal hemorrhoids.

69. The most common cause of urinary obstruction in older males is

a. benign prostatic hyperplasia.
b. tumor.
c. infection.
d. prostatitis.

70. If, following a urethral bulking injection of silicone polymers (Macroplastique), the patient develops urinary retention, the recommended intervention is

a. oxybutynin.
b. aspiration of bulking material.
c. indwelling catheter.
d. intermittent catheterization.

71. Which type of imaging is generally the test of choice for identification of the specific type of fecal incontinence that a patient has?

a. X-ray
b. CT scan
c. anal endoscopic sonography
d. MRI

72. If a patient with stress incontinence has been doing Kegel exercises but still finds she experiences occasional slight incontinence when she coughs or sneezes, the nurse should recommend the use of

a. the "knack."
b. anticholinergics/antimuscarinics.
c. adult diapers.
d. urethral plug.

73. If a female patient complains of new onset of urinary incontinence, which of the following medications may be implicated?

a. stool softener (Colace)
b. thyroid hormone, levothyroxine
c. antidiabetic medication, metformin
d. alpha blocker, doxazosin (Cardura)

74. Which of the following is the most common complication after midurethral sling surgery to correct stress incontinence?

a. infection
b. urinary retention
c. cystocele
d. erosion of mesh into the urethra

75. If a patient is taking mirabegron (Myrbetriq) for treatment of overactive bladder, which of the following should be routinely assessed?

a. platelet count
b. glucose
c. blood pressure
d. WBC count

76. Which of the following is a contraindication to the use of an internal bowel management system?

a. diabetes
b. clotting disorder
c. neurological disease
d. heart disease

77. If urinary incontinence is associated with atrophic vaginitis, treatment may include

a. anticholinergic/antimuscarinic drugs.
b. muscle relaxant.
c. topical estrogen cream or vaginal ring.
d. oral estrogen.

78. What dietary modification is most indicated to help patients control fecal incontinence?

a. increased fiber
b. decreased fiber
c. limited fruit and vegetables
d. fluid restriction

79. If, when adjusting the amplitude for pelvic floor electrical stimulation, the anal wink is absent, this indicates

a. a normal response.
b. nontherapeutic stimulation.
c. the need for increased ramping.
d. the need to increase the on/off to a 2:1 ratio.

80. If a patient has been wearing a pessary but has developed chronic constipation associated with the pessary, the BEST solution is to

a. stop using the pessary.
b. take stool softeners.
c. change to a different size or type of pessary.
d. modify the diet to add more fluids and fiber.

81. The internal fecal management system should be used consecutively for no more than

a. 29 consecutive days.
b. 20 consecutive days.
c. 15 consecutive days.
d. 7 consecutive days.

82. If a post-menopausal patient has a vaginal balloon (Eclipse system) inserted to control fecal incontinence, the patient should be advised to remove the device for cleaning

a. monthly.
b. every 3 weeks.
c. every 2 weeks.
d. every week.

83. When reviewing a patient's management of clean intermittent catheterization, which of the following may indicate increased risk of complications?

a. carrying out intermittent catheterization 3 times daily
b. having a urinary output of 1300 mL per day
c. draining a volume of 200 to 350 mL per catheterization
d. emptying the bladder completely with each catheterization

84. The saline infusion test is given to assess capacity to retain stool by

a. triggering peristalsis.
b. flushing the rectum.
c. softening the stool.
d. simulating diarrhea.

85. If a patient with Parkinson's disease has increasing urinary incontinence, has fallen 3 times in recent months, suffers from depression, and exhibits functional decline, these problems would be best categorized as

a. co-morbidities.
b. geriatric syndromes.
c. disabilities.
d. incidental disorders.

86. What is the normal functional capacity of the bladder?

a. 200 to 300 mL
b. 300 to 400 mL
c. 400 to 600 mL
d. 600 to 800 mL

87. If a family member complains that an 80-year-old patient with multiple health problems (including arthritis) repeatedly urinates on the floor during the night on the way to the bathroom, which is down the hall, the best solution is likely

a. bedside commode.
b. catheterization.
c. fluid restriction in the evening.
d. adult diapers.

88. If, as part of a bowel-training program, the patient has daily scheduled defecation, what is the BEST time to schedule a bowel movement?

a. first thing in the morning after arising
b. at bedtime
c. 2 hours after a meal
d. 20 to 30 minutes after a meal

89. If a patient has developed urinary incontinence and has been researching all different treatment options and comes with a list of questions for the physician, the type of coping strategy this exemplifies is

a. cognitive adaptation.
b. behavioral adaptation.
c. emotion-focused adaptation.
d. avoidance/denial.

90. If a patient is undergoing the balloon (50 mL) expulsion test to assess defecatory disorders, and the patient requires 4 minutes to expel the balloon, this indicates

a. normal defecation.
b. hyperactive bowel.
c. dyssynergic defecatory muscle action.
d. decreased rectal capacity.

91. If an outbreak of *Clostridioides difficile* has resulted in 20 patients in a medical-surgical unit becoming infected and developing severe diarrhea, the breakdown in process that likely caused the outbreak is related to

a. ventilation.
b. handwashing.
c. housekeeping.
d. food handling.

92. Which of the following is likely to have the greatest impact on a patient's access to quality healthcare?

a. socioeconomic status
b. age and gender
c. race/ethnicity
d. place of residence

93. The most important factor in ensuring compliance with the treatment regimen is

a. education.
b. follow-up.
c. therapeutic relationship.
d. cost.

94. Which of the following is an example of functional incontinence?

a. the patient must strain to initiate urine flow and often leaks urine
b. the patient has impaired mobility and often cannot get to the toilet in time
c. the patient tends to leak urine when engaging in strenuous exercise
d. the patient experiences sudden intense urge to urinate and leakage of urine

95. If a 76-year-old female patient complains of nocturnal enuresis but denies having any problem during the daytime, the likely contributing cause is

a. urinary tract infection.
b. nocturnal confusion.
c. medication-associated sphincter impairment.
d. nocturnal polyuria.

96. Overactive bladder in males is most often associated with

a. cancer.
b. dementia.
c. bladder outlet obstruction.
d. smoking.

97. If a patient with urinary incontinence shows the nurse a small notebook that lists all the available toilets in the shopping area of the town, this is an example of

a. toilet mapping.
b. obsessive behavior.
c. risk mitigation.
d. self-care.

98. Strategies for defensive urination include

a. restricting fluid intake prior to activities to decrease urination.
b. urinating on a scheduled basis and before activities.
c. urinating and then waiting for a moment and urinating again.
d. wearing absorbant pads to contain urinary leakage.

99. When assessing a patient's manual dexterity and ability to handle self-care, which of the following activities may be used to assess fine motor skills?

a. lifting the arm from the lap and placing on a table
b. flexing and extending the elbow
c. picking up pencils from a table top and placing in a cup
d. raising the arms over the head while holding weights

100. If a 4-year-old male patient has developed retentive encopresis with leakage of stool, the primary interventions are

a. psychological counseling.
b. reward system.
c. stool softeners and laxatives.
d. scheduled toileting and dietary changes.

101. When assessing a patient for reversible causes of urinary incontinence using the PRAISED mnemonic, the D stands for

a. diuretic use.
b. dehydration/delirium.
c. diapers.
d. dementia.

102. If a patient with severe urge incontinence is learning to manage urgency and feels a strong urge to urinate, the patient should

a. walk slowly to the bathroom.
b. rush to the bathroom.
c. sit and wait until the urge passes.
d. sit on the toilet but try to withhold urination briefly.

103. As part of the bowel diary, the patient is provided a Bristol stool form in order to

a. help to quantify the amount of stool.
b. keep tract of the time and date of defecation.
c. help to identify the type of stool passed.
d. correlate diet with defecation times.

104. The most common type of urinary incontinence in long-term care facilities is

a. stress.
b. overflow.
c. functional.
d. urge.

105. Reflex incontinence is urinary leakage that

a. occurs without a warning sensation.
b. is accompanied by pain.
c. is preceded by feeling of urgency.
d. occurs in response to abdominal pressure.

106. Normal micturition is controlled by the

a. spinal cord.
b. bladder.
c. central nervous system.
d. urinary sphincters.

107. If a patient is learning pelvic floor exercises to increase muscle strength, for the first week or two, the patient should aim to be able to tighten and hold for

a. 1 second.
b. 5 seconds.
c. 10 seconds.
d. 15 seconds.

108. For a patient with dementia who forgets where the bathroom is and doesn't recognize the bathroom if the door is shut, resulting in periodic urinary incontinence, the best solution is likely

a. adult diapers.
b. prompted voiding.
c. bladder training
d. habit training.

109. In a healthy person, the normal frequency of urination during waking hours is every

a. 1 to 2 hours.
b. 2 to 3 hours.
c. 1 to 4 hours.
d. 2 to 6 hours.

110. If a patient complains that it takes at least 60 seconds to initiate urinary flow, as part of assessment the nurse considers that the normal duration is

a. 15 seconds.
b. 30 seconds.
c. 45 seconds.
d. 60 seconds.

111. A patient is considered to have chronic constipation if the patient has bowel movements fewer than

a. 5 times per week.
b. 4 times per week.
c. 3 times per week.
d. 2 times per week.

112. If a patient needs to increase fiber in the diet, which of the following provides the most concentrated form of dietary fiber?

a. whole grain bread
b. fresh fruits
c. fresh vegetables
d. unprocessed wheat bran

113. Prompted voiding is appropriate for a patient having

a. <2 episodes of urinary incontinence in 12 hours.
b. <4 episodes of urinary incontinence in 12 hours.
c. <6 episode of urinary incontinence in 12 hours.
d. <8 episodes of urinary incontinence in 12 hours.

114. Bisacodyl laxative tablets are classified as

a. stimulants.
b. prokinetic agents.
c. osmotic agents.
d. lubricants.

115. Which of the following may increase intestinal fluid secretion and liquid stools?

a. dairy products
b. starchy foods
c. caffeine
d. spicy foods

116. Upon the digital rectal exam for a male patient, a hard lump is felt in the prostate, likely indicating

a. normal prostate.
b. a tumor.
c. hyperplasia.
d. prostatitis.

117. If a bedbound patient is incontinent of frequent loose stools and wears adult diapers but has developed incontinence-associated skin damage, the best solution is likely

a. fecal containment device.
b. more frequent cleansing of skin with soap and water.
c. using underpads only to allow air to reach skin.
d. changing diapers every 2 hours.

118. When utilizing habit training for a patient with urinary incontinence and toileting is scheduled every 3 hours, what is the best response to a patient who has the urge to urinate in 2.5 hours?

a. ask the patient to try to wait 5 minutes before urinating
b. ask the patient to try to wait 15 minutes before urinating
c. ask the patient to try to wait 30 minutes before urinating
d. advise the patient to go ahead and urinate

119. If the nurse notes an itchy red oozing rash in the labial folds, under abdominal rolls, in the underarms, and under the breasts of a very obese patient, this most likely indicates

a. intertriginous dermatitis.
b. contact dermatitis.
c. cellulitis.
d. mechanical irritant dermatitis.

120. The most common psychiatric comorbidity with urinary incontinence is

a. generalized anxiety disorder.
b. depression.
c. bipolar disease.
d. obsessive-compulsive disorder.

Answer Key and Explanations

Continence Care

1. A: Moisture-barrier pastes are ointments with powder added to improve absorption and make them more durable and solid, providing a thick skin barrier. Many are zinc oxide-based, making them somewhat difficult to remove. Mineral oil is often used to remove the paste. Some paste products now on the market are transparent so the skin can be monitored. Pastes are frequently used over denuded or excoriated tissue to absorb exudate and protect from drainage, urine, or feces, so they are used for both perianal and periwound tissues. Pastes are usually reapplied with each dressing/disposable diaper change without being completely removed.

2. D: About 3 to 4 pints of liquid, including digested food, bile, and digestive enzymes, travel through the small intestine to the colon each day. The colon absorbs more than 90% of the fluid as the stool traverses the bowel. Undigested food takes only about 2 hours to reach the colon, but 2 to 5 days to reach the rectum, allowing time for reabsorption. The urge to defecate is caused when the stool travels from the sigmoid colon to the rectum. The rectosigmoid area provides storage. Eating stimulates contractions in the descending and rectosigmoid colon.

3. C: Phase I: Filling/storing is triggered by emptying the bladder. Neurotransmitters in the brain signal the detrusor muscle to relax and the bladder to expand, drawing urine from the kidney and ureters. When the bladder reaches capacity (8 to 16 ounces), nerves send a signal back to the brain. Voluntarily tightening the external sphincter muscles retains the urine. Phase II: Emptying occurs when the nervous system signals the voiding reflex, and spinal nerves contract the detrusor muscle and relax internal sphincter muscles, allowing urine to flow to the urethra. Relaxing external sphincter muscles allows urination.

4. C: Type 3. The Bristol Stool Form is given to people keeping a bowel diary.

- *Type 1* is separate small, hard lumps of stool that are difficult to pass
- *Type 2* is sausage-shaped, lumpy stool
- *Type 3* is sausage-shaped and lumpy, but with cracks on the surface
- *Type 4* is long, smooth, soft, snake-like stool
- *Type 5* is soft blobs of stool that are easily passed and have clear-cut edges
- *Type 6* is mushy, fluffy pieces of stool with uneven ragged edges
- *Type 7* is watery stool that is entirely liquid with no solid pieces

5. B: Postinfectious irritable bowel syndrome is a chronic bowel inflammation that develops in some people after acute enteritis, characterized by altered bowel habits, usually with chronic diarrhea and abdominal pain. About 2/3 of those with IBS have predominately diarrhea, while a fourth alternate between constipation and diarrhea, and the remaining have primarily constipation. Onset of symptoms is often abrupt. Symptoms often persist for years, with 40% still reporting symptoms after 6 years. Treatment is usually with antidiarrheals and a low fiber diet.

6. A: Rectoceles (rectal prolapses) can cause chronic constipation and difficulty in passing stool because of weakening of the muscles, contributing to fecal incontinence. Untreated, rectoceles can cause inflammation, ulceration, and fistula formation. Pessaries may reduce the prolapse. Surgical repair may not correct all symptoms, especially underlying damage to the muscles, and can result in surgical trauma to the rectum or sphincters, adding to the risk of incontinence. Rectoceles occur when the muscles between the wall of the vagina and rectum weaken and the rectum prolapses or protrudes into the back wall of the vagina.

7. B: While some fecal material may leak through fistulae, the primary cause of fistula-associated incontinence is inflammation and tissue damage. Fistulas involving the anus, rectum, or vagina, and the perineal tissue can result in damage to intestinal and pelvic floor muscles, nerves, and sphincters. Anorectal fistulas, the most common type, usually result from an abscess and may have one or more tunnels connecting the rectum and the skin around the anus. Fistulas may also result from trauma, disease, or radiation.

8. D: With MS, the myelin sheath and underlying nerve fibers in the brain, eyes, and spinal cord are damaged or destroyed, sometimes affecting nerves that control bowel movements, causing constipation and fecal incontinence. With PD both voluntary and involuntary muscle control may be compromised, sometimes resulting in loss of sphincter control and fecal incontinence. MD is a group of genetic disorders that cause progressive weakening and atrophy of muscles. Fecal incontinence is a frequent problem with some types of MD: ALS affects the motor neurons, resulting in muscle atrophy and weakness, sometimes causing incontinence.

9. D: Q-tip test measures mobility and axis position of the urethra to assess urinary incontinence in women.

Procedure:

- The patient lies in supine position.
- A cotton swab (Q-tip), sterile and lubricated with anesthetic gel, is inserted through the urethra to the bladder and then pulled back to the bladder neck.
- Supine, the patient strains as though urinating. The angle of the swab is measured when straining and again when resting.
- Standing, the patient again strains, and the angles are measured.
- A positive result is a Q-tip angle of 30°or more at maximal straining, indicating urethral hypermobility.

10. A: Provocative stress maneuver (urinary cough test) is a noninvasive test to determine if coughing will cause urinary stress incontinence in women. The test is done with the woman in supine position. Follow this procedure.

- The patient, with a full bladder, lies in a supine position with legs apart and coughs multiple times. Leakage of urine confirms stress incontinence.
- The patient then stands with one leg on stool and holds a pad or paper towels over the perineum and coughs. A wet stain confirms stress incontinence.

11. C: The mini-mental state exam (MMSE) requires the patient to carry out specified tasks.

- Counting backward from 100 by 7s or spelling "world" backward
- Remembering and later repeating the names of 3 common objects
- Naming items as the examiner points to them
- Providing the location of the examiner's office, including city, state, and street address
- Repeating common phrases
- Copying a picture of interlocking shapes
- Following simple 3-part instructions, such as picking up a piece of paper, folding it in half, and placing it on the floor

12. D: Anal manometry measures the pressure of the sphincter muscles, the degree of sensation in the rectum, and whether the neural reflexes that control normal bowel movements are intact. Anal wink (anocutaneous reflex), reflexive contraction of the anus in response to gentle stroking or stimulation of the skin around the rectum, and bulbocavernosus reflex, reflexive contraction of the anus in response to natural or electrical stimulation of the bulbocavernosus muscle of the penis, are used to determine if there is an interruption or defect in the reflex arc. Endoanal ultrasound is used to diagnose perianal fistulas and abscesses and to assess sphincter damage.

13. A: Foods that cause gas include cabbage, broccoli, kale, onions, turnips, brussel sprouts, asparagus, dried beans, fish, eggs, and strong cheeses. Foods that cause diarrhea or loosening of stool include apple juice, prune juice, fresh fruit, raw vegetables, spicy foods, and fried foods. Foods that cause constipation or thickening of stool include applesauce, bananas, cheese, creamy peanut butter, potatoes, rice, pasta, and marshmallows. Foods that cause obstruction include dried fruits, fruits with skin, nuts, popcorn, whole corn, bean sprouts, celery, and large servings of raw fruits or vegetables.

14. C: Underwear soaked with overflow down legs is estimated to equal 30 to 60 mL volume of incontinence. A bladder diary is kept for 3 to 5 days and includes all urinations and incontinence.

- Time of urination.
- Amount of urination estimated (small, medium, or large) or measured.
- Fluid intake (amount and time).
- Estimate of incontinence (A small volume of less than 30 mL is enough to wet underwear. A moderate volume of 30 to 60 ml is enough to soak underwear with overflow down the legs. A large volume of more than 60 mL is usually enough to soak clothes and run onto floor or furniture.)
- Characterization of incontinence by activity and sensation of urge.

15. B: Anal sphincter electromyography (EMG) assesses muscle contractions to determine if the sphincter muscles are contracting properly. Drugs such as muscle relaxants and both cholinergic and anticholinergic preparations can affect the outcome of the test. This is the procedure.

- With the patient lying on the left side, insert a small lubricated sponge or plug electrode into the anal canal. Alternately, needle electrodes may be used.
- The patient must lie still during the procedure, or the results will be affected.
- The electrical activity of the anal sphincter muscles is recorded on a computer screen while the patient tightens the muscles, then relaxes them and pushes.

16. C: The normal specific gravity of urine is 1.015 to 1.025 with a pH of 4.5 to 8 (average 5 to 6). Urine should be pale yellow or amber, and clear or slightly cloudy. Odor should be slight. Bacteria may give urine a foul odor, depending on the organism, and some foods, such as asparagus, may cause odor. Urine should be free of sediment, glucose, ketones, protein, blood, bilirubin, and nitrates. Urobilinogen ranges from 0.1 to 1 unit.

17. A: During a 24-hour pad test, the pads are weighed before use, and when damp, are sealed in plastic bags and stored. At the end of the 24-hour period, the pads are weighed to determine the total volume of urine lost through incontinence. A shorter version of the test requires the patient to drink 500 mL of liquid, apply a pre-weighed incontinence pad after a half hour, and then engage in some mild to moderate exercise or activity for an hour. Then the pad is weighed to determine the degree of incontinence.

18. D: Cystometry assesses bladder capacity and pressure, including how full the bladder is when the urge to urinate is felt. Electromyography measures activity of the muscles in and around the urethral sphincter. Uroflowmetry measures the flow rate of urine, including the speed of urination and the volume. Pressure flow study measures the amount of bladder pressure that is needed to urinate and the flow rate at different pressures. Leak point pressure measures the bladder pressure at the point where leakage of urine occurs.

19. A: A reduced Valsalva leak point pressure indicates stress incontinence. Valsalva Leak point pressure (VLPP) measures the pressure at which bladder pressure overcomes urethral resistance without contraction of the detrusor muscle of the bladder wall. Use this procedure to check.

- Insert a 6 to 10 Fr. microtip pressure transducer catheter into the bladder.
- Insert rectal probe to monitor intraabdominal pressure.
- The patient sits or stands during the testing.
- Instill the bladder with saline or contrast material at 50 ml min to total of 200 ml.
- Ask patient (sitting or standing) to make a progressive Valsalva motion, bearing down with a closed glottis or coughing, until incontinence.

20. B: When fitting a pessary, a finger should be able to pass easily between the vaginal wall and the pessary. Pessaries are plastic or silicone removable prosthetic devices that are placed in the vagina for management of pelvic muscle support defects, such as cystocele and rectocele. Fitting a pessary may require trial and error to arrive at the correct size and style. The type of pessary is determined by the problem the pessary is intended to correct and the type of muscle weakness or prolapse present. The largest comfortable pessary is the optimum choice for effectiveness.

21. A: Chronic pelvic pain syndrome of unknown etiology (unknown cause or origin) is characterized by persistent or recurrent episodes of pelvic pain that is associated with urinary, sexual, bowel, or gynecological dysfunction, despite lack of evident infection or other pathology. The pain must be continuous or recurrent for 6 months or more. In males, it is often associated with perineal (including anal) and penile pain (often referred to as chronic prostatitis). The distribution and intensity of pain can vary considerably from one individual to another and may involve many different organs and structures.

22. C: Anticholinergics, such as oxybutynin or tolterodine, reduce urinary frequency and incontinence is patients with MS. Almost all MS patients develop difficulty with urination, including frequency, urgency, and incontinence. Some may respond to dietary modification, including avoidance of caffeine or other substances that cause diuresis, such as tea and alcohol. Scheduled voiding may be helpful, but some patients must control incontinence with intermittent straight catheterization every few hours, especially as muscles become increasingly weak and spasticity increases with progression of the disease.

23. D: The average age for menopause is 51. When menopause occurs, ovaries no longer produce eggs, ovulation and menstruation stop, and hormone levels of estrogen and progesterone fall. Estrogen maintains the lining of the bladder and the urethra and stimulates the flow of blood to the pelvic area. As levels of estrogen begin to drop with menopause, the muscles are less well-nourished and the lining of the bladder and urethra may become dry and irritated. The sphincter muscles may lose tone as well.

24. A: Obesity is a primary factor in developing urinary incontinence because of increased stress on muscles, which causes them to weaken and stretch. The increased abdominal mass exerts direct pressure on the bladder. Diuretics may contribute to existing urinary dysfunction, because increased urinary flow stimulates bladder contractions. HPV may result in cervical cancer or genital warts. Oral contraceptives reduce the risk of stress and urgency incontinence as well as overactive bladder because the hormones have a protective effect.

25. D: Social function includes support from family or friends, the need for a caregiver, financial resources, mistreatment or abuse, the ability to drive, and the presence of advance directives. Psychological function includes anxiety, worry, grief, and depression. Those with depression may be at increased risk of physical disability or may neglect self-care. Sensory function includes presence of cataracts, glaucoma, myopia, presbyopia, astigmatism, macular degeneration, or eye disorders that make it difficult for people to read medication labels or perform self-care. Hearing should be evaluated in both ears for hearing deficits and waxy buildup in the ear canals.

26. A: The environmental factor that may most contribute to incontinence in a person with reduced mobility is distance from the bathroom or difficult access to the bathroom, such as when the bathroom is on the second floor. In this case, a urinal (male) or a portable commode should be placed within easier access. Rugs in the hallway and poor lighting may slow the person and increase risk of falls. Toilets should be raised to the appropriate level for the person, with arm supports or grab rails, to facilitate getting on and off the toilet.

27. C: Artificial sweeteners (aspartame, saccharine) are bladder irritants. Other bladder irritants include

- Caffeine, which occurs naturally in coffee beans, tea leaves, and cocoa beans, is added to many soft drinks, and is found in chocolate drinks, candy, and many drugs (Excedrin, Anacin, Fiorinal), by increasing detrusor muscle contractions, resulting in urinary urgency and frequency.
- Citrus foods, such as orange juice, and many other highly acidic fruits.
- Spicy foods, such as Mexican or Chinese food, horseradish, and chili peppers.

28. D: "The knack," a preventive use of Kegel exercises, is using precisely-timed muscle contractions to prevent stress incontinence. It is "the knack" of squeezing up before bearing down. Women learn to contract the pelvic floor muscles right before and during events that usually cause stress incontinence. For example, if a woman feels a cough or sneeze coming, she immediately contracts the pelvic floor muscles and holds until the stress event is over. This contraction augments support of the proximal urethra, reducing the amount of displacement that usually takes place with compromised muscle support, thereby preventing incontinence.

29. A: "Quick flicks" help to treat urinary incontinence by increasing contractility. This procedure utilizes Kegel (pelvic floor) exercises. The patient rapidly contracts and relaxes the pelvic floor muscles, usually in sets of 10 or 20, repeated 10 times, so each set includes up to 200 quick flicks. "Slow squeeze," contracting over a count of 2 to 4, holding for 3 to 4 seconds, and then relaxing is used to increase endurance. Most people with incontinence should do both types of exercises.

30. C: The most important factor in decreasing constipation is to increase dietary fiber and fluids. Exercise also helps to reduce constipation by increasing motility, but some people may be physically limited in their ability to exercise. Stool softeners may also help reduce constipation, but are not a substitute for dietary management. Laxatives should be avoided, as overuse may result in a cycle of constipation and diarrhea.

31. C: Liquid stool often leaks around a fecal impaction, resulting in incontinence. The pressure of the stool often causes hemorrhoids to become engorged. Fecal impaction occurs when the hard stool moves into the rectum and becomes a large, dense, immovable mass that cannot be evacuated, even with straining, usually as a result of chronic constipation. In addition to abdominal cramps and distention, the person may feel intense rectal pressure and pain, accompanied by a sense of urgency to defecate. Nausea and vomiting may also occur.

32. D: Food sources of soluble fiber include bananas, starches (potatoes, bread), cheese, dried beans, nuts, apples, oranges, and oatmeal. Soluble fiber dissolves in liquids to form a gel-like substance. This is one reason liquids are so important in conjunction with fiber in the diet. Soluble fiber slows the movement of stool through the gastrointestinal system. Insoluble fiber changes little with the digestive process and increases the speed of stool through the colon, so too much can result in diarrhea. Food sources of insoluble fiber include seeds, skins of fruits and vegetables, and nuts. Oat bran contains both soluble and insoluble fiber.

33. B: Defecation should be scheduled for 20 to 30 minutes after a meal, when there is increased motility. Scheduled defecation is usually at the same time daily, but for some people it is done only 3 to 4 times weekly, depending on individual bowel habits. Stimulation is necessary. Drinking a cup of hot liquid may work, but initially many require rectal stimulation with a gloved finger. Some people require rectal suppositories, such as glycerin, but stimulus suppositories or enemas should be avoided if possible. The patient should be sitting upright with knees elevated slightly, if possible, and leaning forward during defecation.

34. D: The initial step in controlling occasional urinary incontinence is scheduled urination, in which the patient is asked to urinate at scheduled intervals. Fluids should not be limited, as dehydration can impair wound healing. Foley catheters should be avoided if at all possible because they pose considerable risk of urinary and systemic infections. Anticholinergic medications can be used if other efforts fail and if incontinence is due to muscle spasms.

35. B: Black, tarry stools may occur from digested blood from the upper gastrointestinal tract or from iron supplements, black dye (licorice), or Pepto-Bismol. Clay-colored stools may indicate lack of sufficient bile or use of antidiarrheals, such as Kaopectate. Orange stools may be caused by medications (Rifadin, Rimactane) or beta-carotene in pills or foods, such as apricots, carrots, sweet potatoes, pumpkin, and mangoes. Green stools may be caused by leafy vegetables or green dye in foods. With diarrhea, it's possible that the bile didn't break down when the stool moved quickly through the colon, causing a green color. Bright yellow stools may indicate bile obstruction.

36. C: Desmopressin at bedtime reduces urinary production for 5 to 6 hours. Antidepressants, such as Imipramine, relax the bladder and tighten the urethral sphincter, and anticholinergics (such as oxybutynin) reduce instability of the detrusor muscle. Tamsulosin (Flomax) may reduce nocturnal enuresis in males with benign prostatic hypertrophy. Other treatments for nocturnal enuresis include behavior modifications such as bladder training, scheduled urination, fluid restriction, and dietary modifications. Conditioning therapy with enuresis alarms may be helpful, especially for primary nocturnal enuresis.

37. C: A test to determine correct size of vaginal weights is to begin inserting the lightest weight cone into the vagina, requiring the pelvic muscles to tighten to hold it in place. If the patient can hold it in place for one minute, progress to the next higher weight, increasing the weights incrementally to determine the heaviest weight that can be held for one minute. Exercise with the vaginal weights is usually done two times a day for 15 minutes until the heaviest weight can be held.

38. D: Bladder training, a behavioral therapy, has an improvement rate of about 75% for urge incontinency, so it is the treatment of choice. Scheduled urination should be done, gradually increasing time between urinations, along with strategies to delay urination. People who have dementia or caregivers may need prompted urination in order to maintain a schedule. Medications are usually given only if behavioral therapy is unsuccessful. Surgical treatment is not recommended for urge incontinence. Reducing caffeine and other bladder irritants may reduce contractions.

39. C: Because all treatments can have adverse effects, treatment for BPH usually begins conservatively with medications. Alpha-blockers (such as tamsulosin and alfuzosin) relax the prostatic and bladder neck muscles to facilitate urination, and 5-alpha-reductase inhibitors (such as finasteride and dutasteride) help prevent further enlargement and may shrink the prostate. If medical treatments do not provide relief of symptoms, then prostatectomy or less invasive procedures, such as high-intensity focused ultrasound, transurethral needle ablation, or microwave and thermotherapy (water-induced) may be indicated.

40. A: The treatment of choice for a male with detrusor sphincter dyssynergia (most commonly related to spinal cord injury or multiple sclerosis) is insertion of a urethral stent (UroLume), because the procedure is less invasive than an external sphincterectomy, and urethral stents are reversible. Long-term catheterization poses the risk of infection and urethral trauma, and urinary diversion poses more risks. Detrusor sphincter dyssynergia occurs when involuntary contractions of the detrusor muscle coincide with involuntary contraction of the external urethral sphincter, resulting in obstruction that may cause vesicourethral reflux, hydronephrosis, sepsis, kidney stones, and renal failure.

41. C: Conservative treatment for DHIC is most common and includes bladder training with scheduled urination, or prompted urination, and if necessary, Credé maneuver and double voiding. Anticholinergics may worsen DHIC: Other treatment includes diet modifications to eliminate bladder irritants. While intermittent clean catheterization may be needed, long-term catheterization increases the risk of infection. Detrusor hyperactivity with impaired contractile function (DHIC) is characterized by overactive detrusor contractions during the storage phase but underactive contractions during urination, resulting in both frequency and residual urine in bladder. It is common with neurological impairment from trauma or with diseases such as Parkinson's or multiple sclerosis.

42. A: A fecal pouch is an external pouching devise that is applied to intact skin to protect the anus and perianal area from contamination and irritation caused by fecal incontinence. The fecal pouch can manage a volume of ≤500 mL of liquid or semi-liquid stool. The bag is attached with adhesive for a secure fit and is changed every 24 to 72 hours or if leakage occurs. A fecal containment system is used with >500 mL of liquid or semi-liquid stool daily. Disposable underwear is used for ambulatory patients. Refastenable briefs may not be adequate to prevent maceration of skin.

43. C: The best solution for helping a patient with mild dementia remember to urinate is an alarm system that sets off a bell, beep, or flashing light at regularly set intervals. While disposable underwear may also be useful, the patient should be encouraged to maintain scheduled urination to reduce incontinence and risk of skin irritation. Catheterization should be avoided, because of risk of trauma and infection and difficulty in self-care. A telephone reminder may not be practical as a long-term solution.

44. D: A penile clamp should be released on a regular schedule of every 2 hours to prevent complications. Penile clamps apply pressure around the penis to compress the urethra and prevent incontinence. It is clamped about halfway down the penis shaft and has soft foam on the inside of the clamp. The clamp is released at least every 2 hours to prevent circulatory restriction and to allow for urination. It is very important that the clamp not be placed too tightly, because it can cause strictures, skin breakdown, or even necrosis.

45. C: The urethral plug (such as the FemSoft TM) may prevent stress incontinence during strenuous exercise. The plugs are for one-time use and must be removed and replaced every 3 to 4 hours. An alternative is the external urethral patch (such as the Impress SoftpatchTM), but it may be more easily dislodged. Absorbent pads contain fluids but don't prevent incontinence. Valved catheters are intended for long-term use and are usually changed about every 28 days. Tampons are intended for menstrual flow, but some women find that tampons provide pressure against the urethra, preventing mild incontinence.

46. B: Biofeedback aims to increase sensory perception and control of the muscles of defecation. A sensor is placed in the rectum or around the external sphincters. An electromyograph sensor or intraanal manometric pressure probe may be inserted into the anus. Strength training uses manometry to measure pressure of the anal sphincters during contraction and relaxation. Coordination exercises are done to ensure that the internal and external anal sphincters are working in concert. The person receives instant feedback from a visual or auditory response regarding the ability to sense fullness in the rectum and to contract and relax the sphincter muscles.

47. D: Phosphate (Fleet) enemas come prepackaged for one-time use with about 120 mL of solution. They stimulate contractions and, because they are hypertonic, draw fluid back into the intestines. Frequent use can result in hyperphosphatemia (>4.5 mEq/L) when too much phosphate is absorbed into the bloodstream. Symptoms include tachycardia, muscle cramping, hyperreflexia, tetany, nausea, and diarrhea. Hypocalcemia (<8.2 mg/dL) can also result. Symptoms include tetany, tingling, seizures, altered mental status, and ventricular tachycardia.

48. A: With augmentation cystoplasty, a section of the colon is removed, shaped, and sutured into the bladder wall to expand the bladder capacity. With the sling procedure for women, abdominal, donor, or synthetic tissue is placed under the urethra, acting like a hammock and compressing the urethra to prevent leakage. With TVT, a mesh tape is placed under the urethra, acting like a hammock. With retropubic suspension, the urethra and bladder neck are repositioned and secured.

49. B: While catheters at home may be reused after washing and drying, sterilization is more effective in preventing infection. At-home sterilization can be done by boiling the catheters and equipment for 10 minutes, pouring off liquid, and placing catheters in sealable plastic bags. An alternate method is to place the clean and dry catheters and equipment on a paper towel in the microwave with a glass of water and to microwave on high for 6 minutes. The glass of water in the microwave will provide steam.

50. A: The amplitude of the electrical current must be sufficiently strong to elicit the anal wink, or it will be ineffective. The patient may experience pain if ramping (speed at which the current reaches the muscles) is too fast. The frequency rate may vary, but is usually set at 50 Hz to increase strength for stress incontinence and 13 Hz to relax muscles for urge incontinence. The ratio of on to off for electrical stimulation should be 1:1 (minimal) to 1:2 (most common), for example 5 seconds with current on and 10 seconds with current off.

51. B: For female patients undergoing anal sphincteroplasty, the most common problem in the postoperative period is difficulty urinating, and this may continue for days or even weeks while healing takes place. The ability to urinate is evaluated after surgery, and if patients are unable to initiate flow, then they may require an indwelling catheter or learn to carry out clean intermittent catheterization if able to do so until they can urinate independently.

52. A: The first indication that a patient may develop fecal incontinence is flatus incontinence. If a patient is unable to prevent the loss of flatus through the anus, over time some stool may begin to be expelled with the flatus, and the sphincter may continue to weaken. Therefore, with any indication of flatus incontinence, the patient should undergo testing to determine if interventions are appropriate in order to prevent further deterioration.

53. D: If a patient is diagnosed with detrusor external sphincter dyssynergia (DESD), the nurse expects the treatment plan to include clean intermittent catheterization. Patients with DSD have suprasacral lesions that result in inability to voluntarily control urination as well as loss of bladder-sphincter coordination although the reflex arc remains intact, so the detrusor muscle contracts when the bladder is full, but the sphincter may contract at the same time.

54. A: If a patient has quit smoking and has been chewing sugar free gum and snacking on carrots, nuts, and celery all day to control cravings but has developed recurrent diarrhea, the most likely cause of the diarrhea is sugar free chewing gum. Many sugar free chewing gums contain sorbitol, which can cause flatus and has a laxative effect, especially if the person is chewing multiple pieces of gum throughout the day. Additionally, people tend to swallow more air while chewing gum, which increases bloating.

55. B: If using ultrasound scanning to decrease obsessive toileting for a patient with overactive bladder the patient should be urged to delay urination if the bladder volume is less than 100 mL to 150 mL. Patients with obsessive toileting often have volumes of 50 to 75 mL. It's important to engage the patient in the scanning process, showing them the results and explaining what that means. If the volume is small, the patient should be encouraged to try to delay voiding for at least 15 minutes.

56. C: Patients with fecal incontinence often try to self-manage for years before discussing the problem with healthcare providers primarily because they feel shame and embarrassment about the incontinence. Some patients may also be unaware that there are options to control incontinence. Healthcare providers should directly ask patients if they have had any problem with urinary and/or fecal incontinence, especially those at increased risk, such as patients with diabetes.

57. B: The most common cause of fecal incontinence in females is obstetric trauma, especially if associated with perineal tears (third and fourth degree), instrumental delivery, breach delivery, or epidural anesthesia. Those at increased risk include primiparas and grand multiparas and those who receive oxytocin during the second stage of labor to speed labor and delivery.

58. A: When treating urge urinary incontinence with pelvic floor electrical stimulation, the frequency rate, pps/Hz, should be set at 13 pps/Hz. If treating stress incontinence, 50 pps/Hz is utilized. The on/off time refers to the ratio of time the muscle is exposed to current and is at rest. This on/off ratio is usually 1:2, but at no times should the on time exceed the off time because inadequate recovery time could lead to muscle fatigue.

59. D: If a patient is undergoing bladder training and is trying to resist the urge to urinate for one-hour periods but feels a strong urge to urinate after 40 minutes, the patient should be advised to practice distraction techniques, such as relaxation and deep breathing exercises. As preparation for bladder training, the patient should practice various distraction techniques to determine which are most effective. Often, the strong urge to urinate will pass if the patient is able to avoid urinating because the volume of urine is likely small with frequent voiding.

60. C: If the urinalysis is positive for leukocyte esterase, this usually indicates pyuria because it indicates the presence of white blood cells (an indication of infection). Vaginal secretions and trichomonas infection may give an inaccurate test result, and high protein and vitamin C levels may provide a false negative. Other indications of a urinary infection include presence of nitrite and RBCs (bleeding results from irritation caused by infection). If a urea-splitting organism is present, the pH may increase.

61. A: The pessary that is most appropriate for treatment for cystocele stress urinary incontinence is the Gehring with knob. The knob applies pressure to the cystocele. Gehrung pessaries are U-shaped and provide support under the bladder and keep the uterus from descending. The Gehring pessary is more successful than many pessaries in keeping the cystocele from slipping out of place. When inserted, the pessary should provide a bridge to hold the bladder in place.

62. B: Smoking increases the risk of urinary incontinence, especially stress incontinence, and the more the patient smokes, the more the impact, especially if the person smokes more than 20 cigarettes daily. While smoking can worsen all forms of incontinence, it is believed that the cough associated with smoking tends to increase the risk of early development of stress incontinence through weakening the pelvic floor muscles. Smoking also increases the risk of developing bladder cancer.

63. D: Reservoir incontinence is associated with decreased colonic or rectal capacity, which may occur with chronic rectal ischemia or irritable bowel syndrome. Reservoir incontinence may also occur after previous surgical repair of the rectum as well as from prolapse of pelvic organs into the rectal vault. Those with irritable bowel syndrome may have decreased tolerance to capacity. In some cases, increased capacity (such as with megacolon) may also lead to incontinence because evacuation may be inadequate, leading to impaction.

64. C: Proctography (AKA defecography) is the test used to determine the amount of fecal material the rectum can accommodate and how effectively the stool is expelled. For the procedure, the patient must drink a container of 500 mL of barium liquid about an hour prior to imaging. With the patient in left Sims position, a catheter is inserted into the rectum and barium (sometimes thickened with other materials) injected until the patient has the urge to defecate at which time the patient is seated on a special commode beside a fluoroscope which takes x-ray images during defecation. For females, a small catheter is inserted into the vagina and about 5 mL of barium injected to help to distinguish the organs on the films.

65. D: For patients with fecal incontinence, the most troubling physical effect is generally urgency. Patients are often fearful of going out in public or socializing with others because they fear that they will experience urgency and be unable to find a bathroom in time to avoid incontinence. The feeling of urgency may come on very abruptly, so the patient often experiences anticipatory anxiety that interferes with the ability to socialize with others.

66. B: Simethicone (Mylicon, Gas-X) may relieve flatus incontinence and can be purchased by patients OTC. Beano, an enzyme-based product, may also help to reduce gas. Patients should also be educated about foods that produce gas, such as beans and cruciferous vegetables (cabbage, Brussels sprouts, cauliflower, broccoli), and carbonated beverages. Lactose, found in dairy products, may also cause gas in some individuals.

67. C: If, during an interview, older patients fail to mention urinary incontinence, it is often because they believe incontinence is a natural part of aging, a common myth. Therefore, they often delay seeking medical help for the problem until it is severe enough to seriously impact their lives. Others may believe that there is no effective treatment. Some may feel embarrassed about urinary incontinence and associate it with hygiene problems, preferring to use absorbent pads rather than to face the shame of discussing the problem.

68. B: If a patient with no previous fecal incontinence has developed a sudden onset of slow leakage of stool and a feeling of rectal discomfort, the patient should be assessed for fecal impaction. With impaction, a hard mass of stool forms in the colon or rectum and the body attempts to compensate by decreasing absorption of liquid from the stool above the impaction, and this liquid stool then often leaks around the impaction. If the impaction is in the rectum, the pressure may impair sphincter control, resulting in leakage.

69. A: The most common cause of urinary obstruction in older males is benign prostatic hyperplasia (BPH). The symptoms do not necessarily correlate with the size of the enlargement. Typical indications include frequency and urgency, difficulty initiating stream, weak or intermittent stream, and leakage of urine. Risk factors for BPH include older age, family history of prostatic hyperplasia, diabetes, heart disease, beta blockers, and obesity.

70. D: If, following a urethral bulking injection of silicone polymers (Macroplastique), the patient develops urinary retention, the recommended intervention is intermittent catheterization. Urinary retention is common for the first few days until swelling subsides, but an indwelling catheter may put too much pressure on the implants and result in leakage of urine. For intermittent catheterization, a small gauge catheter should be utilized to ensure that trauma is minimized. Macroplastique is very viscous so it is injected with a high-pressure injection gun into the mid-urethra at the 6, 10, and 12 o'clock positions.

71. C: Anal endoscopic sonography is generally the imaging test of choice for identification of the specific type of fecal incontinence that a patient has and has often replaced electromyography, which required that needles be inserted into the muscles of the sphincter. Anal endoscopic sonography is able to identify the type of damage that has occurred to the sphincters. Patients are generally asked to take a colon prep to ensure the rectum is empty prior to the ultrasound.

72. A: Since the patient has only occasional stress incontinence and has been doing Kegel exercises, the gerontological nurse should recommend the use of the "knack," which is precisely-timed contractions of the pelvic floor muscles immediately before and during a stressful event (such as a cough or sneeze) to prevent incontinence. This maneuver helps to provide support to the urethra. The knack is effective for mild to moderate urinary incontinence and can decrease incontinence by 70% to 98%.

73. D: If a female patient complains of new onset of urinary incontinence, the medication that may be implicated is the alpha blocker (alpha-adrenergic antagonists), doxazosin (Cardura), which can cause reduced bladder outlet resistance. Alpha blockers may increase incontinence in females by up to 5 times. Other medications often implicated in incontinence include clonidine, methyldopa, antipsychotics, diuretics, ARBs, CCBs, ACEIs, estrogens, hypnotics, antidepressants, and hydroxychloroquine.

74. B: The most common complication after midurethral sling surgery to correct stress incontinence is urinary retention. Some patients also may experience new onset of urgency. These symptoms usually recede over time. Less common complications include erosion of the mesh into the urethra, urinary obstruction, and infection. Pain should be mild to moderate after the procedure. Severe pain may indicate hematoma or injury to muscle or nerve.

75. C: If a patient is taking mirabegron (Myrbetriq) for treatment of overactive bladder with urgency, frequency, and urinary leakage, the patient's blood pressure should be routinely assessed because the most common adverse effect of mirabegron is hypertension. Other adverse effects may include cold and flu symptoms, dry mouth, back and joint pain, headaches, cystitis, and UTI. While mirabegron works similarly to oxybutynin, it tends to have fewer adverse effects and may be used for patients with glaucoma.

76. B: A clotting disorder is a contraindication to the use of an internal bowel management system, especially if the patient is taking anticoagulants or antiplatelet drugs. The internal balloon may cause irritation to the tissue with bleeding, and bleeding can also occur if the internal portion is inadvertently pulled out. Other contraindications include inadequate sphincter tone, anal stenosis, ischemic mucosa, hemorrhoids (severe), and fecal impaction.

77. C: If urinary incontinence is associated with atrophic vaginitis, treatment may include topical estrogen cream or vaginal ring (Estring), which provides a steady dose of estradiol over a 90-day period after insertion. Vaginal cream is applied with a slide-in applicator and is used daily for several weeks and then three times weekly. Oral estrogen is not advised because of adverse effects associated with the oral preparation. Atrophic vaginitis is common in postmenopausal women because the vaginal wall begins to atrophy because of the diminished supply of estrogen.

78. A: While causes for fecal incontinence may vary, the dietary modification that is most indicated to help patients control the fecal incontinence is increased fiber. This may be accomplished through dietary fiber (whole grains, fruits, vegetables) or the use of high fiber bulking agents, such as psyllium (Metamucil), but patients must have an adequate fluid intake or constipation may occur. The patient may benefit from a regular toileting program. In some cases, fecal incontinence is associated with excessive use of laxatives.

79. B: If, when adjusting the amplitude for pelvic floor stimulation, the anal wink is absent, this indicates nontherapeutic stimulation; that is, the current is not resulting in contraction of the sphincter, which likely indicates denervation of the pelvic floor. In that case, electrical stimulation of the pelvic floor muscles will not be a successful treatment, and other alternatives must be considered.

80. C: If a patient has been wearing a pessary but has developed chronic constipation associated with the pessary, the best solution is to change to a different size or type of pessary. Patients often need to change pessaries 2 to 3 times before the correct fit and comfort level is achieved, so patients should be encouraged to report any problems that arise, such as constipation, which usually occurs when the pessary applies too much pressure to the rectum.

81. A: The internal fecal management system should be used for no more than 29 consecutive days. Indications for the internal fecal management system include fecal incontinence (4-5/12 hrs) of liquid to semi-liquid stool, expectation of liquid stool for more than 3 days, and possible contamination of wound from fecal material. Patients who are completely ambulatory are not good candidates because they will likely not retain the device.

82. D: If a post-menopausal patient has a vaginal balloon (Eclipse system) inserted to control fecal incontinence, the patient should be advised to remove the device for cleaning weekly. If women are pre-menopausal, they should remove the device daily during menses. The vaginal balloon, which has tubing attached, is inserted into the vagina like a tampon, with the tube hanging out of the vagina. A pump is attached to the tubing to inflate and deflate the balloon. The balloon is deflated when the patient needs to defecate.

83. A: When reviewing a patient's management of clean intermittent catheterization, carrying out intermittent catheterization only 3 times daily may indicate increased risk of complications. Intermittent catheterization should be done 4 to 6 times daily in order to ensure that the bladder volume does not exceed 400 mL. Infrequent catheterization may result in bladder distention and stagnant urine, increasing the risk of infection. The bladder should be completely emptied with each catheterization, and total urine volume should not fall below 1200 mL/day.

84. D: The saline infusion test is given to assess capacity to retain stool by simulating diarrhea. A small catheter is inserted into the rectum and taped in place and then the patient is seated on a commode and warm saline solution is infused at the rate of 60 mL/min while the patient is instructed to tighten the sphincters and hold the fluid as long as possible. At the first leakage of 15 mL or more, the volume of liquid infused is noted. Usually about 800 mL to 1500 mL of NS is infused and a patient with normal sphincter control can usually hold most of the liquid.

85. B: If a patient with Parkinson's disease has increasing urinary incontinence, has fallen 3 times in recent months, suffers from depression, and exhibits functional decline, these problems would best be categorized as geriatric syndromes, which is the occurrence of disease along with age-related conditions. Diseases that are often associated with geriatric syndromes also include diabetes mellitus, peripheral arterial disease, cerebrovascular disease, and Alzheimer's. Common problems associated with geriatric syndromes include cognitive impairment, urinary incontinence, depression, falls, fractures, and functional decline.

86. C: The normal functional capacity of the bladder is 400 to 600 mL. Beyond that, the bladder may become distended and uncomfortable, and the risk of overflow urinary incontinence increases. As the bladder fills, the detrusor muscle of the bladder wall stretches, allowing the bladder to expand. The internal muscle layer of the bladder, the urothelium, contains sensory processes. The sphincter mechanism controls the flow of urine into the urethra, which is about 3 to 4 cm long in females and 20 cm in males.

87. A: If a family member complains that an 80-year-old patient with multiple health problems repeatedly urinates on the floor during the night on the way to the bathroom, which is down the hall, the best solution is likely a bedside commode as this appears to be functional incontinence. Because of the arthritis, the patient probably must move slowly and is, therefore, unable to hold the urine for the time it takes to reach the bathroom.

88. D: The best time for scheduled evacuation is 20 to 30 minutes after a meal because eating stimulates motility. The scheduled time (usually daily but may be 3-4 times weekly, depending on individual habits) should be at the same time each day, so work hours or activities should be considered. Stimulation may include drinking hot liquid or rectal stimulation (inserting a gloved, lubricated finger into the anus and running it around the rim of the sphincters). The best position for defecation is upright and leaning forward with knees elevated slightly. The patient should massage the abdomen, strain, and attempt to tighten abdominal muscles and relax sphincters if possible.

89. B: If a patient has developed urinary incontinence and has been researching all different treatment options and comes with a list of questions for the physician, the type of coping strategy this exemplifies is behavioral adaptation because the patient is actively seeking solutions to mitigate the condition. Those utilizing behavioral adaptation are interested in finding the cause of a problem and dealing directly with the cause and likely to feel in control and informed.

90. C: If a patient is undergoing the balloon (50 mL) expulsion test to assess defecatory disorders, the normal time to expel the balloon is 1 minute. If the patient requires more than 3 minutes, this is an indication of dyssynergic defecatory muscle action. For this test, a balloon is inserted into the rectum and filled with 50 mL of air or water and then the patient is asked to expel the balloon and the time needed to expel is recorded.

91. B: If an outbreak of *Clostridioides difficile* has resulted in 20 patients in a medical-surgical unit becoming infected, the breakdown in process that likely caused the outbreak related to inadequate handwashing. *C. difficile* is commonly spread through spores in the feces which contaminate the hands of healthcare workers and transfer to environmental surfaces. Alcohol-based hand scrubs do not adequately kill the spores, so when infections with *C. difficile* are suspected or confirmed, then handwashing should be done consistently with soap and water.

92. A: The patient's socioeconomic status is likely to have the greatest impact on a patient's access to quality healthcare. Patients with low income may not be able to afford insurance or may have insurance with a very large deductible or restrictions in coverage. Patients may be unable to qualify for Medicaid because of assets or because their income is slightly above the cutoff level. Patients may be unable to afford prescription drugs or prescribed treatments, and this may negatively impact their health outcomes.

93. C: While all of these (education, cost, follow-up) are important, the most important factor in ensuring compliance with the treatment regimen is the therapeutic relationship between the patient and the healthcare provider. If the patient feels trust, and the healthcare provider takes the time to discuss patient concerns (such as convenience and cost) and explain both the need for the treatment and the consequences of failing to comply, some of the problems that arise with compliance may be avoided.

94. B: If a patient has impaired mobility and often cannot get to the toilet in time, this is an example of functional incontinence, which can include any physical or psychological problem that interferes with the patient's ability to self-toilet even though the person may be aware of the need to do so. Possible physical problems that may result in functional incontinence include impaired vision, environmental barriers (stairways, poor lighting, long distance), cognitive impairment, musculoskeletal disorders, and neurological disorders.

95. D: If a 76-year-ld female patient complains of nocturnal enuresis but denies having any problem during the daytime, the likely contributing cause is nocturnal polyuria. Water excretion tends to shift with older age with about 33% (and up to 50% in some people) of urine production occurring during the night coupled with decreased release of antidiuretic hormone during the night. Also, during the daytime, fluid tends to increase in extracellular spaces, but this fluid is released more quickly into the bloodstream during the night when the patient is in supine position.

96. C: Overactive bladder (OAB) in males is most often associated with bladder outlet obstruction. However, this is rarely the case with females because of a much shorter urethra. Bladder outlet obstruction in males is most often caused by benign prostatic hyperplasia, which compresses the urethra and causes difficulty with urination and increased risk of urinary infection, which further impairs urination. About half of those with BPH also have detrusor overactivity. BPH primarily affects males over age 60.

97. A: If a patient with urinary incontinence shows the nurse a small notebook that lists all of the available toilets in the shopping area of the town, this is an example of toilet mapping. The patient wants to be sure to know where all bathrooms are located in case of urgent need. Patients attempting to deal with urinary incontinence without medical assistance often result in multiple strategies to manage incontinence, including restricting activities outside of the home because of the fear of incontinence.

98. B: Strategies for defensive urination include urinating on a scheduled basis, such every 2 hours and before activities that may increase incontinence, like exercise. If urinary incontinence is severe, patients may find they need to urinate more and more frequently in order to prevent or control incontinence, and this can become not only time-consuming but exhausting and burdensome. Patients often combine this strategy with fluid restriction, increasing the risk of urinary infection, which in turn worsens incontinence.

99. C: The activity that may be used to assess fine motor skills includes picking up pencils from a table top and placing the pencils in a cup. Other assessments include the box and block test in which blocks are moved from one section of a box to another section and the 9-hold peg test in which pegs are picked up, placed in a peg-board, removed, and returned to the original container. The activities are timed.

100. D: If a 4-year-old male patient has developed retentive encopresis with leakage of stool, the primary interventions are scheduled toileting and dietary changes. While positive reinforcement (praise, rewards) and stool softeners may help to encourage the child to cooperate and to facilitate bowel function, scheduling toileting after meals and increasing fiber in the diet are essential. The child may also need to increase fluid intake and decrease intake of food high in fat and simple carbohydrates as these slow the movement of fecal material through the digestive tract.

101. B: Dehydration/Delirium. PRAISED mnemonic for reversible causes of urinary incontinence:

P	Pharmaceuticals/Psychological problems
R	Restricted mobility/Retention
A	Atrophic urethritis/Vaginitis
I	Infection (urinary), symptomatic
S	Stool impaction
E	Excessive urinary output (from endocrine or cardiovascular disease, excessive fluid intake, pedal edema)
D	Dehydration/Delirium (and other confusion-inducing states)

102. A: If a patient with severe urge incontinence is learning to manage urgency and feels a strong urge to urinate, the patient should walk slowly to the bathroom. Rushing to the bathroom often results in increasing the contractions of the bladder muscles, so the patient is more likely to have an episode of incontinence. Initially, when a patient is trying to avoid rushing, the patient should be situated near a bathroom to reduce anxiety and encourage compliance.

103. C: As part of the bowel diary the patient is provided a Bristol stool form (which contains pictures and descriptions) in order to help to identify the type of stool passed:

- Type 1: Separate small hard lumps of stool that are difficult to pass.
- Type 2: Sausage-shaped lumpy stool.
- Type 3: Sausage-shaped and lumpy but with cracks on the surface.
- Type 4: Long, smooth, soft, snake-like stool.
- Type 5: Soft blobs of stool that are easily passed and have clear-cut edges.
- Type 6: Mushy, fluffy pieces of stool with uneven ragged edges.
- Type 7: Watery stool that is entirely liquid with no solid pieces.

104. D: The most common type of urinary incontinence in long-term care facilities is urge incontinence. Urge incontinence is often associated with impaired cognition or physical impairment and is common with neurological disorders, such as MS, SCI, CVA, and Parkinson's disease. Some things may serve as triggers, for example, a patient may feel increased urge to urinate when approaching the patient's room or bathroom, a condition referred to "key-in-the-lock" because the person unconsciously associates the action of returning to the room or bathroom with urinating.

105. A: Reflex incontinence is urinary leakage that occurs without a warning sensation when the bladder contracts involuntarily (often with a large volume of urine excreted) without any feeling of urgency because of damage to the nerves. Reflex incontinence may be associated with MS, SCI, or other neurological disorder. Reflex incontinence is similar to urge incontinence even though the patient lacks the sensation of urgency, so treatment for reflex incontinence is similar.

106. C: Normal micturition is controlled by the central nervous system, including an area in the pons referred to as the pontine micturition center, the central relay. While micturition is an autonomic reflex, urinating is under voluntary control mediated by the spine and brain. Contraction of the bladder is controlled by the sacral micturition center (S2-S4). The cerebral cortex inhibits the sacral micturition center. Therefore, neurological disorders or damage to different parts of the brain may affect different aspects of micturition.

107. B: If a patient is learning pelvic floor exercises to increase muscle strength, for the first week or two, the patient should aim to be able to tighten and hold for 5 seconds. Exercises should be done at least 3 times daily. They may be done, for example, while lying down in the morning and evening and while sitting midday.

- *1-2 weeks:* Tighten 1 second, relax 5. Repeat 10 times.

  Then tighten 5 seconds and relax 10. Repeat 10 times.

- *3-4 weeks:* Tighten 5-10 seconds and relax 10. Repeat 20 times.
- *5-6 weeks:* Tighten 8-10 seconds and relax 10. Repeat 20 times.

108. B: For a patient with dementia who forgets where the bathroom is and doesn't recognize the bathroom if the door is shut, resulting in periodic urinary incontinence, the best solution is likely prompted voiding and assisting the patient to locate the bathroom. Placing a picture of a toilet on the bathroom door or painting the bathroom a distinctive color may help the patient to recognize the bathroom, but the patient may still need prompting because of the dementia.

109. D: In a healthy person, the normal frequency of urination during waking hours is every 2 to 6 hours, and can vary depending on such factors as ambient temperature, activity level, and fluid intake. If, however, a person continually urinates every 2 hours, this would be considered abnormal, as most people urinate between 4 and 10 times in a 24-phour period. Children urinate more frequently than adults because the capacity of their bladders is less.

110. A: If a patient complains that it takes at least 60 seconds to initiate urinary flow, as part of assessment the nurse considers that the normal duration is 15 seconds. Urine hesitancy is common in males, especially those with prostatic hyperplasia. Other causes may include surgical trauma, childbirth, infection, neurological impairment (MS, CA), disorder of bladder muscle, shy bladder syndrome (inability to urinate when others are present), tumor, or medications (anticholinergics/antimuscarinics, antidepressants.

111. C: A patient is considered to have chronic constipation if the patient has bowel movements fewer than 3 times per week. Constipation is usually characterized by a number of different complaints: hard stool, need to strain, feeling of rectal fullness and blockage, need to splint, and inability to completely empty rectum. The most common form of constipation is normal-transit constipation in which the stool traverses the colon in the usual time but is hard and difficult to pass.

112. D: If a patient needs to increase fiber in the diet, unprocessed wheat bran provides the most concentrated form of dietary fiber as it contains 40% fiber. Bran may be added to other foods, such as cereals, ice cream, fruit, and puddings, and is often combined with applesauce and prune juice (which has a laxative effect) in a mixture and given to patients (4 to 5 tablespoons) daily in order to prevent constipation. Processed bran in cereals is less effective.

113. B: Prompted voiding is appropriate for a patient having <4 episodes of urinary incontinence in 12 hours (during waking hours). Prompted voiding includes verbal toileting reminders and positive feedback. Prompted voiding begins with a 3-day trial period during which patients are asked if they are wet or dry and then checked and feedback provided. Patients are then asked if they want to use the toilet and if refusing to do so, are prompted 3 times. The trial period helps to assess the patients' awareness of continence and the need to urinate.

114. A: Bisacodyl laxative tablets are classified as stimulants, which stimulate nerve endings to increase intestinal motility. Stimulants generally work within 1 to 6 hours but should not be taken long-term or frequently because they may cause damage to the bowel and result in electrolyte imbalances. Simulants should not be taken with warfarin (may decrease effectiveness of warfarin) or with dairy products or antacids (may decrease effectiveness of the stimulant).

115. C: Caffeine may increase intestinal fluid secretion and liquid stools, which may increase incidence of fecal incontinence. Patients should be advised to avoid fluids and foods high in caffeine, such as caffeinated beverages (tea, coffee, cola drinks) and chocolate. Foods high in starch (pasta, potatoes, sweets, beans) and cruciferous vegetables (Brussels sprouts, cabbage) and spicy foods may increase production of gas, which can also increase the risk of flatus-associated fecal incontinence.

116. B: Upon the digital rectal exam for a male patient, a hard lump is felt in the prostate, likely indicating a tumor. The exam may be carried out with the patient in left lateral Sims position or standing and leaning forward against an examining table. The prostate should extend about 1 cm into the rectum and be about 3.5 cm in width. The prostate should feel smooth and firm. If a lump is felt, then a biopsy is usually done to confirm presence of tumor/malignancy.

117. A: If a bedbound patient is incontinent of frequent loose stools and wears adult diapers but has developed incontinence-associated skin damage (IASD), the best solution is likely a fecal containment device because this prevents fecal material from coming in contact with the skin and allows air to circulate. IASD is more common with fecal or mixed fecal/urinary incontinence than with just urinary incontinence because of the enzymes found in the fecal material.

118. C: When utilizing habit training for a patient with urinary incontinence and toileting is scheduled every 3 hours, the best response to a patient who has the urge to urinate in 2.5 hours is to ask the patient to try to wait 30 minutes (the entire 3 hours) before urinating. Often the urge to urinate will subside if the patient waits for a period of time. With habit training, the established schedule for urinating is based on the patient's own pattern of urination.

119. A: If the nurse notes an itchy red oozing rash in the labial folds, under abdominal rolls, in the underarms, and under the breasts of a very obese patient, this most likely indicates intertriginous dermatitis. This often develops in areas of the skin that lack adequate circulation of air and where the skin rubs together, causing friction and irritation. Moisture, such as from perspiration, urine, or feces may worsen the condition. Infection is common, especially with yeast, such as *Candida*, but bacteria and other types of fungi may be implicated.

120. B: The most common psychiatric comorbidity with urinary incontinence is depression, which is commonly found in older adults, especially those with chronic illness. Up to 25 to 50% of those with urinary incontinence experience sexual dysfunction (often because they are afraid of experiencing incontinence during coitus), and many feel that the quality of their lives is negatively impacted. They may experience feelings of shame and humiliation and actively avoid social situations, further adding to their isolation and feelings of depression.

How to Overcome Test Anxiety

Just the thought of taking a test is enough to make most people a little nervous. A test is an important event that can have a long-term impact on your future, so it's important to take it seriously and it's natural to feel anxious about performing well. But just because anxiety is normal, that doesn't mean that it's helpful in test taking, or that you should simply accept it as part of your life. Anxiety can have a variety of effects. These effects can be mild, like making you feel slightly nervous, or severe, like blocking your ability to focus or remember even a simple detail.

If you experience test anxiety—whether severe or mild—it's important to know how to beat it. To discover this, first you need to understand what causes test anxiety.

Causes of Test Anxiety

While we often think of anxiety as an uncontrollable emotional state, it can actually be caused by simple, practical things. One of the most common causes of test anxiety is that a person does not feel adequately prepared for their test. This feeling can be the result of many different issues such as poor study habits or lack of organization, but the most common culprit is time management. Starting to study too late, failing to organize your study time to cover all of the material, or being distracted while you study will mean that you're not well prepared for the test. This may lead to cramming the night before, which will cause you to be physically and mentally exhausted for the test. Poor time management also contributes to feelings of stress, fear, and hopelessness as you realize you are not well prepared but don't know what to do about it.

Other times, test anxiety is not related to your preparation for the test but comes from unresolved fear. This may be a past failure on a test, or poor performance on tests in general. It may come from comparing yourself to others who seem to be performing better or from the stress of living up to expectations. Anxiety may be driven by fears of the future—how failure on this test would affect your educational and career goals. These fears are often completely irrational, but they can still negatively impact your test performance.

Elements of Test Anxiety

As mentioned earlier, test anxiety is considered to be an emotional state, but it has physical and mental components as well. Sometimes you may not even realize that you are suffering from test anxiety until you notice the physical symptoms. These can include trembling hands, rapid heartbeat, sweating, nausea, and tense muscles. Extreme anxiety may lead to fainting or vomiting. Obviously, any of these symptoms can have a negative impact on testing. It is important to recognize them as soon as they begin to occur so that you can address the problem before it damages your performance.

The mental components of test anxiety include trouble focusing and inability to remember learned information. During a test, your mind is on high alert, which can help you recall information and stay focused for an extended period of time. However, anxiety interferes with your mind's natural processes, causing you to blank out, even on the questions you know well. The strain of testing during anxiety makes it difficult to stay focused, especially on a test that may take several hours. Extreme anxiety can take a huge mental toll, making it difficult not only to recall test information but even to understand the test questions or pull your thoughts together.

Effects of Test Anxiety

Test anxiety is like a disease—if left untreated, it will get progressively worse. Anxiety leads to poor performance, and this reinforces the feelings of fear and failure, which in turn lead to poor performances on subsequent tests. It can grow from a mild nervousness to a crippling condition. If allowed to progress, test anxiety can have a big impact on your schooling, and consequently on your future.

Test anxiety can spread to other parts of your life. Anxiety on tests can become anxiety in any stressful situation, and blanking on a test can turn into panicking in a job situation. But fortunately, you don't have to let anxiety rule your testing and determine your grades. There are a number of relatively simple steps you can take to move past anxiety and function normally on a test and in the rest of life.

Physical Steps for Beating Test Anxiety

While test anxiety is a serious problem, the good news is that it can be overcome. It doesn't have to control your ability to think and remember information. While it may take time, you can begin taking steps today to beat anxiety.

Just as your first hint that you may be struggling with anxiety comes from the physical symptoms, the first step to treating it is also physical. Rest is crucial for having a clear, strong mind. If you are tired, it is much easier to give in to anxiety. But if you establish good sleep habits, your body and mind will be ready to perform optimally, without the strain of exhaustion. Additionally, sleeping well helps you to retain information better, so you're more likely to recall the answers when you see the test questions.

Getting good sleep means more than going to bed on time. It's important to allow your brain time to relax. Take study breaks from time to time so it doesn't get overworked, and don't study right before bed. Take time to rest your mind before trying to rest your body, or you may find it difficult to fall asleep.

Along with sleep, other aspects of physical health are important in preparing for a test. Good nutrition is vital for good brain function. Sugary foods and drinks may give a burst of energy but this burst is followed by a crash, both physically and emotionally. Instead, fuel your body with protein and vitamin-rich foods.

Also, drink plenty of water. Dehydration can lead to headaches and exhaustion, especially if your brain is already under stress from the rigors of the test. Particularly if your test is a long one, drink water during the breaks. And if possible, take an energy-boosting snack to eat between sections.

Along with sleep and diet, a third important part of physical health is exercise. Maintaining a steady workout schedule is helpful, but even taking 5-minute study breaks to walk can help get your blood pumping faster and clear your head. Exercise also releases endorphins, which contribute to a positive feeling and can help combat test anxiety.

When you nurture your physical health, you are also contributing to your mental health. If your body is healthy, your mind is much more likely to be healthy as well. So take time to rest, nourish your body with healthy food and water, and get moving as much as possible. Taking these physical steps will make you stronger and more able to take the mental steps necessary to overcome test anxiety.

Mental Steps for Beating Test Anxiety

Working on the mental side of test anxiety can be more challenging, but as with the physical side, there are clear steps you can take to overcome it. As mentioned earlier, test anxiety often stems from lack of preparation, so the obvious solution is to prepare for the test. Effective studying may be the most important weapon you have for beating test anxiety, but you can and should employ several other mental tools to combat fear.

First, boost your confidence by reminding yourself of past success—tests or projects that you aced. If you're putting as much effort into preparing for this test as you did for those, there's no reason you should expect to fail here. Work hard to prepare; then trust your preparation.

Second, surround yourself with encouraging people. It can be helpful to find a study group, but be sure that the people you're around will encourage a positive attitude. If you spend time with others who are anxious or cynical, this will only contribute to your own anxiety. Look for others who are motivated to study hard from a desire to succeed, not from a fear of failure.

Third, reward yourself. A test is physically and mentally tiring, even without anxiety, and it can be helpful to have something to look forward to. Plan an activity following the test, regardless of the outcome, such as going to a movie or getting ice cream.

When you are taking the test, if you find yourself beginning to feel anxious, remind yourself that you know the material. Visualize successfully completing the test. Then take a few deep, relaxing breaths and return to it. Work through the questions carefully but with confidence, knowing that you are capable of succeeding.

Developing a healthy mental approach to test taking will also aid in other areas of life. Test anxiety affects more than just the actual test—it can be damaging to your mental health and even contribute to depression. It's important to beat test anxiety before it becomes a problem for more than testing.

Study Strategy

Being prepared for the test is necessary to combat anxiety, but what does being prepared look like? You may study for hours on end and still not feel prepared. What you need is a strategy for test prep. The next few pages outline our recommended steps to help you plan out and conquer the challenge of preparation.

Step 1: Scope Out the Test

Learn everything you can about the format (multiple choice, essay, etc.) and what will be on the test. Gather any study materials, course outlines, or sample exams that may be available. Not only will this help you to prepare, but knowing what to expect can help to alleviate test anxiety.

Step 2: Map Out the Material

Look through the textbook or study guide and make note of how many chapters or sections it has. Then divide these over the time you have. For example, if a book has 15 chapters and you have five days to study, you need to cover three chapters each day. Even better, if you have the time, leave an extra day at the end for overall review after you have gone through the material in depth.

If time is limited, you may need to prioritize the material. Look through it and make note of which sections you think you already have a good grasp on, and which need review. While you are studying, skim quickly through the familiar sections and take more time on the challenging parts.

Write out your plan so you don't get lost as you go. Having a written plan also helps you feel more in control of the study, so anxiety is less likely to arise from feeling overwhelmed at the amount to cover.

Step 3: Gather Your Tools

Decide what study method works best for you. Do you prefer to highlight in the book as you study and then go back over the highlighted portions? Or do you type out notes of the important information? Or is it helpful to make flashcards that you can carry with you? Assemble the pens, index cards, highlighters, post-it notes, and any other materials you may need so you won't be distracted by getting up to find things while you study.

If you're having a hard time retaining the information or organizing your notes, experiment with different methods. For example, try color-coding by subject with colored pens, highlighters, or post-it notes. If you learn better by hearing, try recording yourself reading your notes so you can listen while in the car, working out, or simply sitting at your desk. Ask a friend to quiz you from your flashcards, or try teaching someone the material to solidify it in your mind.

Step 4: Create Your Environment

It's important to avoid distractions while you study. This includes both the obvious distractions like visitors and the subtle distractions like an uncomfortable chair (or a too-comfortable couch that makes you want to fall asleep). Set up the best study environment possible: good lighting and a comfortable work area. If background music helps you focus, you may want to turn it on, but otherwise keep the room quiet. If you are using a computer to take notes, be sure you don't have any other windows open, especially applications like social media, games, or anything else that could distract you. Silence your phone and turn off notifications. Be sure to keep water close by so you stay hydrated while you study (but avoid unhealthy drinks and snacks).

Also, take into account the best time of day to study. Are you freshest first thing in the morning? Try to set aside some time then to work through the material. Is your mind clearer in the afternoon or evening? Schedule your study session then. Another method is to study at the same time of day that you will take the test, so that your brain gets used to working on the material at that time and will be ready to focus at test time.

Step 5: Study!

Once you have done all the study preparation, it's time to settle into the actual studying. Sit down, take a few moments to settle your mind so you can focus, and begin to follow your study plan. Don't give in to distractions or let yourself procrastinate. This is your time to prepare so you'll be ready to fearlessly approach the test. Make the most of the time and stay focused.

Of course, you don't want to burn out. If you study too long you may find that you're not retaining the information very well. Take regular study breaks. For example, taking five minutes out of every hour to walk briskly, breathing deeply and swinging your arms, can help your mind stay fresh.

As you get to the end of each chapter or section, it's a good idea to do a quick review. Remind yourself of what you learned and work on any difficult parts. When you feel that you've mastered the material, move on to the next part. At the end of your study session, briefly skim through your notes again.

But while review is helpful, cramming last minute is NOT. If at all possible, work ahead so that you won't need to fit all your study into the last day. Cramming overloads your brain with more information than it can process and retain, and your tired mind may struggle to recall even previously learned information when it is overwhelmed with last-minute study. Also, the urgent nature of cramming and the stress placed on your brain contribute to anxiety. You'll be more likely to go to the test feeling unprepared and having trouble thinking clearly.

So don't cram, and don't stay up late before the test, even just to review your notes at a leisurely pace. Your brain needs rest more than it needs to go over the information again. In fact, plan to finish your studies by noon or early afternoon the day before the test. Give your brain the rest of the day to relax or focus on other things, and get a good night's sleep. Then you will be fresh for the test and better able to recall what you've studied.

Step 6: Take a Practice Test

Many courses offer sample tests, either online or in the study materials. This is an excellent resource to check whether you have mastered the material, as well as to prepare for the test format and environment.

Check the test format ahead of time: the number of questions, the type (multiple choice, free response, etc.), and the time limit. Then create a plan for working through them. For example, if you have 30 minutes to take a 60-question test, your limit is 30 seconds per question. Spend less time on the questions you know well so that you can take more time on the difficult ones.

If you have time to take several practice tests, take the first one open book, with no time limit. Work through the questions at your own pace and make sure you fully understand them. Gradually work up to taking a test under test conditions: sit at a desk with all study materials put away and set a timer. Pace yourself to make sure you finish the test with time to spare and go back to check your answers if you have time.

After each test, check your answers. On the questions you missed, be sure you understand why you missed them. Did you misread the question (tests can use tricky wording)? Did you forget the information? Or was it something you hadn't learned? Go back and study any shaky areas that the practice tests reveal.

Taking these tests not only helps with your grade, but also aids in combating test anxiety. If you're already used to the test conditions, you're less likely to worry about it, and working through tests until you're scoring well gives you a confidence boost. Go through the practice tests until you feel comfortable, and then you can go into the test knowing that you're ready for it.

Test Tips

On test day, you should be confident, knowing that you've prepared well and are ready to answer the questions. But aside from preparation, there are several test day strategies you can employ to maximize your performance.

First, as stated before, get a good night's sleep the night before the test (and for several nights before that, if possible). Go into the test with a fresh, alert mind rather than staying up late to study.

Try not to change too much about your normal routine on the day of the test. It's important to eat a nutritious breakfast, but if you normally don't eat breakfast at all, consider eating just a protein bar. If you're a coffee drinker, go ahead and have your normal coffee. Just make sure you time it so that the caffeine doesn't wear off right in the middle of your test. Avoid sugary beverages, and drink enough water to stay hydrated but not so much that you need a restroom break 10 minutes into the test. If your test isn't first thing in the morning, consider going for a walk or doing a light workout before the test to get your blood flowing.

Allow yourself enough time to get ready, and leave for the test with plenty of time to spare so you won't have the anxiety of scrambling to arrive in time. Another reason to be early is to select a good seat. It's helpful to sit away from doors and windows, which can be distracting. Find a good seat, get out your supplies, and settle your mind before the test begins.

When the test begins, start by going over the instructions carefully, even if you already know what to expect. Make sure you avoid any careless mistakes by following the directions.

Then begin working through the questions, pacing yourself as you've practiced. If you're not sure on an answer, don't spend too much time on it, and don't let it shake your confidence. Either skip it and come back later, or eliminate as many wrong answers as possible and guess among the remaining ones. Don't dwell on these questions as you continue—put them out of your mind and focus on what lies ahead.

Be sure to read all of the answer choices, even if you're sure the first one is the right answer. Sometimes you'll find a better one if you keep reading. But don't second-guess yourself if you do immediately know the answer. Your gut instinct is usually right. Don't let test anxiety rob you of the information you know.

If you have time at the end of the test (and if the test format allows), go back and review your answers. Be cautious about changing any, since your first instinct tends to be correct, but make sure you didn't misread any of the questions or accidentally mark the wrong answer choice. Look over any you skipped and make an educated guess.

At the end, leave the test feeling confident. You've done your best, so don't waste time worrying about your performance or wishing you could change anything. Instead, celebrate the successful completion of this test. And finally, use this test to learn how to deal with anxiety even better next time.

Review Video: Test Anxiety
Visit mometrix.com/academy and enter code: 100340

Important Qualification

Not all anxiety is created equal. If your test anxiety is causing major issues in your life beyond the classroom or testing center, or if you are experiencing troubling physical symptoms related to your anxiety, it may be a sign of a serious physiological or psychological condition. If this sounds like your situation, we strongly encourage you to seek professional help.

Online Resources

Due to our efforts to try to keep this book to a manageable length, we've created a link that will give you access to all of your online resources:

mometrix.com/resources719/cccn

It's Your Moment, Let's Celebrate It!

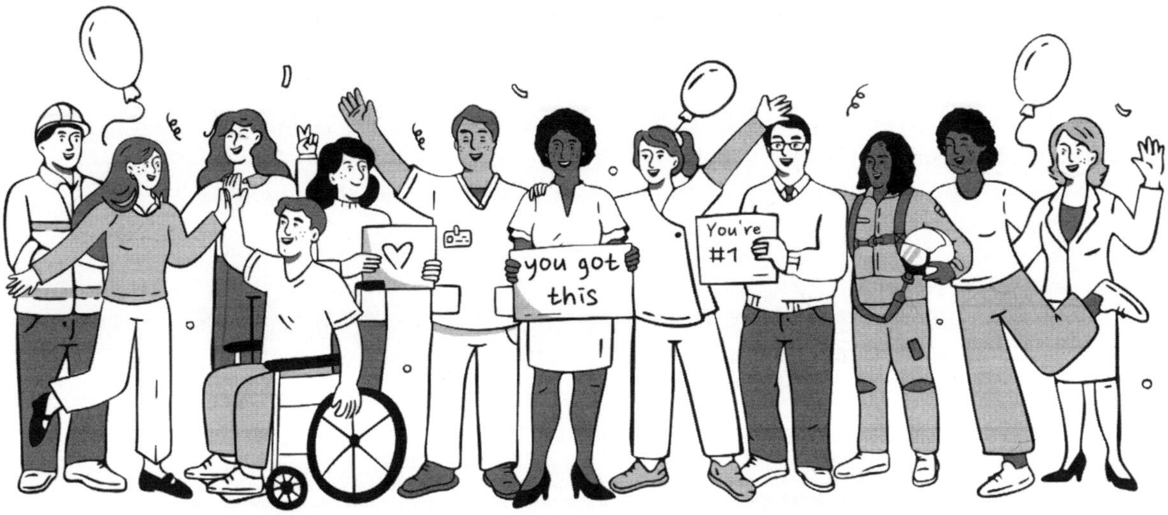

Share your story @mometrixtestpreparation